RC
147
.H6
F73
1982

**FREUDBERG, Frank. Herpes: a complete guide to relief & reassur-
ance. Running Press, 1982. 159p bibl index 82-13303. 12.95 ISBN
0-89471-193-8; 6.95 pa ISBN 0-89471-188-1. CIP**
A very comprehensive and easy-to-understand summary of what is currently known about the diagnosis and management of herpes virus infections. Freudberg is a fine writer with a readable narrative style. The sections
on the immune system and on nutrition are particularly revealing and well
done. The appendix contains an excellent glossary of terms for the unin-
itiated, plus a bibliography and other interesting data relating to the herpes
problem. Brief interviews with people who have contracted herpes help
readers understand the many concerns of afflicted individuals. This informative and well-constructed volume is a welcome addition to the growing
literature on herpes virus, which is now assuming epidemic proportions in
the American public. For all libraries.

LARRY A. JACKSON LIBRARY
Lander College
Greenwood, S. C. 29646

HERPES

A Complete Guide to Relief and Reassurance

Herpes

A Complete Guide to Relief & Reassurance

Frank Freudberg

Introduction by
E. Stephen Emanuel, M.D.

346022

Running Press
Philadelphia, Pennsylvania

JACKSON LIBRARY · LANDER

Copyright ©1982 by Running Press
All rights reserved under the Pan-American
and International Copyright Conventions.
Printed in the United States of America

Canadian representatives: John Wiley & Sons Canada, Ltd.
22 Worcester Road, Rexdale, Ontario M9W 1L1

International representatives: Kaiman & Polon, Inc.
2175 Lemoine Avenue, Fort Lee, New Jersey 07024

9 8 7 6 5 4 3 2 1
Digit on the right indicates the number of this printing.

Library of Congress Cataloging in Publication Data
Freudberg, Frank
Herpes: a complete guide to relief and reassurance
Bibliography:p.
Includes index.
1. Herpes simplex   I. Title
RC147.H6F73   1982   616.95′18   82–13303
ISBN 0–89471–188–1 (paperback)
ISBN 0–89471–187–3 (library binding)

Typography: Paladium by rci
Printed by Port City Press

This book may be ordered from the publisher.
Please include 95 cents postage.

Try your bookstore first.

Running Press
125 South 22nd Street
Philadelphia, Pennsylvania 19103

Table of Contents

Many people provided invaluable assistance to me during the writing of this book—far too many to mention here. But I am particularly grateful for the invaluable contributions of Sam Knox, director of the American Social Health Association, and of its Herpes Resource Center—and for their permission to excerpt liberally from The Helper.

Also, the Philadelphia HELP chapter provided me with continuous support and information, adding greatly to the scope of the project.

Scores of herpesvirus patients selflessly shared their experiences in order to benefit others.

Linus Pauling, twice winner of the Nobel Prize, shared his insight into controlling this enigmatic virus, offering his thoughts about Vitamin C's effects on the human immune system. Thanks also to the Linus Pauling Institute of Science and Medicine for its help.

And finally, I must express my appreciation and thanks to Running Press, without whose advice and counsel this book would not have been as successful.

Introduction

Herpesvirus, once thought of as just a simple, innocuous sore occuring around the lips or nose and associated with a cold, has now become one of America's most dreaded diseases.

Because the lesions are recurrent, the disease has caused havoc in many sexual relationships. I have seen marriages and friendships disrupted because of the fear of catching or spreading the disease. I have heard of men who have developed varying degrees of psychological impotence because of their anxieties about herpesvirus. I have heard women renounce lovemaking because they have contracted the disease—and in my practice I have seen many women deeply anxious, tearful and afraid while awaiting the results of herpesvirus cultures.

Now we are finding herpesvirus to be associated with cervical cancer in women. And it is life-threatening to newborns; if a pregnant woman at term has an active herpes sore around the vaginal area, Caesarean-section delivery is indicated.

The disease is classified as an STD (a sexually transmitted disease) because skin-to-skin contact is the most common method of its spread. We now find, however, that the virus is capable of surviving many hours on in-animate objects and therefore may have additional ways of being con-tracted. The virus is already estimated to be present in tens of millions of Americans—and with a base of that magnitude, its increased spread becomes inevitable.

Many methods of treatment for herpesvirus infection have been tried over the years. Some of these methods have looked quite promising at first, only to be found ineffective or dangerous. Some are still in use, but only because of their effect as placebos—which gives them at least some significance in herpesvirus treatment. A recent new drug, Acyclovir, has come upon the market, but this product shortens the duration of the disease only in the primary attack—and only slightly, at that. Furthermore, it does not affect recurrences at all.

Frank Freudberg and I have done much digging in all of the known aspects of herpesvirus, including anti-viral research, psychological response, ineffective cures, comfort measures, implications in pregnancy and childbirth, the question of cancer, and the management of stress. Our goal is to educate and enlighten the general public, while emphasizing that through awareness and cooperation with one's physician, herpesvirus *can* be effectively managed. We hope this book meets that challenge.

— E. Stephen Emanuel, M.D.
Philadelphia
August, 1982

A Problem That Won't Go Away

1

Herpes Simplex: A New Epidemic

I didn't realize the damn thing was contagious as hell. Who knows how many women I've infected? — HERBERT R.

Herbert L., a 44–year–old advertising executive, lives and works in Wilmington, Delaware. Almost fifteen years ago, when he was single, he was dating several women when he noticed an unusual swelling and several small blisters on his penis.

Herbert: *The doctor examined me for about two seconds, if I remember correctly, and left the room, returning with a huge book—I guess a volume of symptoms and diseases. He thumbed through it for a minute and then just shrugged. "Wild women, right?" he asked me.*

I admitted that I'd been with a few different women lately. "VD, Doc?" I asked him.

"No," he replied, "but one of them gave you that virus." I was confused because to me the word "virus" meant—you know, chills, headache, sore throat; the flu kind of virus. I guess I looked worried, and he almost laughed. "Don't worry about it," he said. "It's just a little virus. It'll go away."

I asked him what I could take for it. "Nothing," he said. "It'll clear up by itself." Then he went on to ask me about my neck, which I had strained playing touch football earlier that summer. He made nothing of the infection. On my way out of the office, almost as an afterthought, I asked, "By the way, what's this infection called?"

He said it was called Herpes progenitalis—and then reminded me not to lift anything heavy on account of my neck. But the name herpes stuck in my head. And every few years I would get an itching sensation and then a little patch of blisters would break out—always at the same place, right on the shaft of my penis, below the head. They'd clear up in a few days, scab over, and that'd be it.

I've had herpes for about fifteen years now, I guess. I never gave it much thought; I was glad that it healed up so quickly, and the subsequent times, the sores were never as bad. But in the last year or two, herpes has been getting a lot of press. Everywhere I go, it's herpes,

herpes, herpes. I started to get a real complex over it. People would talk about herpes, and even though I had read everything I could find about it, I'd play dumb. Then, they'd joke and laugh about it, and I'd join. I really felt like a secret agent—like Typhoid Mary or something . . .

A doctor quickly reads over a lab report, drops it onto his desk, and looks up at a nervous patient. "It's definite," he says. "You have herpes." That scene, or one just like it, happens every day in the United States—more than 1400 times. The Centers for Disease Control in Atlanta estimate that as many as half a million new cases are contracted each year—but other authorities believe the number of new infections to be twice that. No one is sure exactly how widespread genital herspesvirus infections are, but the estimates range from a low of 10 million cases in the United States to a high of 40 million cases and more.* Anywhere from one in five to one in three adults are infected.

The virus particles responsible have been discovered in all kinds of animals, from monkeys to oysters. In humans, sores caused by herpesvirus, called *lesions*, are most commonly found on or around mucous membranes such as the lips or genitals, but can erupt virtually anywhere on the skin surface, as well as in the eyes, nose and brain.

At one end of the scale, the disease can be completely asymptomatic. (By the time they reach age 50, most Americans will have herpesvirus antibodies circulating in their blood—an indication that they have had contact with the disease at least once in their lifetime.) At the other, it can cause brain damage and death. Herpes keratitis, in which herpesvirus attacks the eye, can cause blindness if left unchecked. About 70% of the babies who do become infected will die, and half the survivors suffer damage to the brain or central nervous systems, blindness or other serious impairment. Infants up to about six months of age who contract herpesvirus infections—usually by touching or being touched by someone with an active infection—can also be seriously damaged.

The term *epidemic* comes from the Greek *epi* meaning "on" or "at" and *demos*, "people." An epidemic can establish itself only when a high percentage of the host population is susceptible; and herpesvirus, particularly genital herpesvirus, is now considered an epidemic. The virus is spread only be direct contact. Sores are usually visible, but the "shedding" of viral particles can occur invisibly, before any sores appear. Herpesvirus has been afflicting man for thousands of years, and probably much longer than that. But given today's sexual freedom, it's not difficult to understand

---

* Throughout this book, all estimates of the number of herpesvirus sufferers are approximate. This is because unlike syphilis or hepatitis, new cases of herpesvirus are not required by law to be reported to health officials. Therefore, we have polled a number of experts and authorities and the range of their best estimates is reported here.

A PROBLEM THAT WON'T GO AWAY

why the disease is spreading like the proverbial wildfire. For many people, casual intimacy is a way of life. Sexual contact with friends, co-workers, schoolmates, even absolute strangers is not uncommon. And so, the "pool" of infected persons is constantly increasing. This disease has become the number-one sexually transmitted health problem in the United States and is fast achieving that dubious distinction throughout the rest of the world.

Of course, some people who contract genital herpesvirus never infect anyone else. But there are others who, through ignorance or irresponsibility, infect any number of others. One 30-year-old California woman believed she had contracted herpesvirus from her unfaithful husband. In revenge, she decided to infect as many men as she could. By her own estimate, she infected some twenty-five men a year for three years running, until a psychotherapist helped her see that her behavior was injurious to others, and psychologically self-destructive. If each of the men she infected managed to spread the virus to two other women, then several hundred cases of herpesvirus could be traced to the actions of that one woman.

This is one epidemic not likely to check itself or naturally burn out: the number of infectious people is hardly likely to decrease in the forseeable future, if only because of the increasing number of new cases. But in addition, herpes simplex is a viral disease with no known cure. Herpesviruses are unique parasites that have learned to "hide" where they are inaccesible to the body's natural system of defenses. During its countless ages of evolution, the herpes simplex virus has found a safe niche in the human anatomy where it can succeed in escaping the antibodies despatched to destroy and remove it from the system. Among the greatest obstacles to controlling and managing this condition is the patient's personal reluctance to accept the fact that the virus is in the body to stay—forever. Certain physical and psychological occurrences are known to cause dormant herpesvirus particles to become suddenly active. A new outbreak of herpesvirus can be triggered by a number of factors, including fevers and other illnesses, sunlight, moisture, friction, and—significantly—psychological stress. Later, in Chapter 13, we'll examine different ways to avoid signalling the herpesvirus to awaken from its latent state.

While herpesvirus can create a complex set of physical symptoms, its most taxing effects are generally psychological and emotional. A herpesvirus lesion that appears on the lip (commonly known as a cold sore) is usually painful, sometimes embarrassing, but basically a minor annoyance. Yet move that identical sore onto the penis, vagina, cervix or thighs, buttocks, anus and lower abdomen—and its troublesome characteristics are multiplied a hundredfold, often causing fantastic mental anguish and distress. Patients agree that discussing this recurrently contagious disease with others, particularly a prospective lover, can be a devastating experience. Herpesvirus has been known to wreck marriages, and drive despairing sufferers to suicide. But in most cases, herpesvirus can be managed quite effectively. And to a large extent, the frequency and intensity of recurrences *can* be diminished.

In interviewing people for this book, we've uncovered dozens of myths and misconceptions about herpesvirus infections; most of them concerning genital herpesvirus. Following are a few of the more common ones:

Herpes simplex virus Type I (HSV–I) is the oral variety of the virus, and herpes simplex virus Type II (HSV–II) is the genital variety.

Either of these closely related strains can cause a genital *or* oral infection. Unfortunately, the number of cases of genital herpesvirus is catching up to those of oral herpesvirus, mainly because of the increased popularity of oral sex. Over the past decade the "crossover" rate has soared, and estimates suggest that within the next few years, HSV–I and HSV–II will occur orally and genitally in roughly equal numbers of cases. But according to Dr. Andre Nahmias of Atlanta's Emory University, research has shown that for some reason, herpes simplex Type I, when contracted genitally, is less likely to recur than herpes simplex Type II.

Gay women do not get genital herpesvirus infections.

Not so. The virus invades *cells*, not sexual preferences. A woman with a cold sore on her lip, for example, can transfer the virus particles to her partner's mouth or genitals. (The same applies, of course, to gay men.)

Once people get herpesvirus, they can no longer have sex.

Not so! Sex can still be had whenever one desires. But should a recurrence become evident, a herpesvirus patient should postpone sexual contact.

Men who catch herpesvirus become impotent as a result.

Generally, men rarely suffer periodic impotence (defined as the inability to achieve or maintain an erection) as the result of organic problems. Men who become anxious about sexual performance frequently report periods of transient impotence. Thus, impotence in male herpesvirus patients is most likely the result of anxiety over recurrences, or about sexual self-image in general. Many men have reported that they suffered occasional periods of impotence even before contracting the genital form of the virus.

If one spouse has the virus, his or her mate will eventually get it.

If the couple is careful and practices the methods of hygene and prevention outlined in Chapter 12, there is no reason why the mate ever has to contract herpesvirus. Patients are infectious only periodically, and only during these periods of infectiousness must they assume the responsibility of not spreading the virus particles to the uninfected.

Herpesvirus infections cause cancer in women.

Although women with genital herpesvirus infections do run a statis-

A PROBLEM THAT WON'T GO AWAY

tically greater chance of cervical cancer, there is no documentable proof that the virus *causes* cancer of the cervix. Later, in Chapter 10, we'll examine the apparent connection between herpesvirus and cervical cancer. Women who have herpesvirus are actually *less* likely to die of cervical cancer, because their doctors will have advised them to get Pap smears at least annually—and Pap smears can alert physicians to a pre-cancerous condition long before the disease actually develops. Should cervical cancer ever develop, as it does in some 6 percent of women who contract a genital herpes infection, there is a 100 percent effective cure. Awareness is fundamental to controlling herpesvirus and its more deleterious effects.

Women who have genital herpesvirus can't give birth to healthy children.

If a woman with a concurrent vaginal herpesvirus infection gives birth, chances are good that her infant will contract the virus—and because a newborn's immune system is so rudimentary, death is a likely prognosis. Any infant surviving a herpesvirus infection runs an almost certain chance of blindness, brain damage or injury to the central nervous system. But as we'll see later, effective precautions can make such neonatal infections relatively rare. There are between 20 and 25 million genital herpesvirus patients in the U.S. Yet last year, it is estimated that fewer than 1,000 babies born (out of 3.5 million) suffered from any herpesvirus complication.

Children don't get herpesvirus infectons.

On the contrary, children are *highly* susceptible to the virus, and they can pick it up from towels, toothbrushes, drinking cups, and other inanimate objects handled by anyone with an active infection. Neonates and infants younger than six months are particularly vulnerable because of their immature immune systems.

There is a vaccine for herpesvirus, but it's expensive and accessible only to the very wealthy.

To our knowledge, not true. If such a vaccine existed, it would be effective only in protecting persons who have not yet contracted the virus. Vaccines are preventatives, not cures. Two dangerous, crippling manifestations of herpesvirus *are* treatable: Herpes keratitis (in which the virions attact the eye) and Herpes encephalitis (brain infection). But no form of herpesvirus infection is 100 percent curable.

Of course, great strides in anti-viral and anti-herpes research are being made daily. With the advent of heightened public awareness and increased funding for research, many authorities feel that the development of an effective weapon against this ubiquitous virus is imminent. There is the likelihood that eventually, an anti-viral drug will be developed that can rid the world of herpes. Science *is* getting closer every day, and treatments are becoming more and more effective. But *at this moment*, no such cure exists.

Therefore, herpesvirus sufferers have to concentrate on one simple goal: how to diminish the frequency and intensity of herpesvirus recurrences.

By practicing simple measures of preventive hygiene, the spread of herpesvirus can be dramatically reduced. Throughout, this book offers methods of achieving high levels of nutrition, ways of reducing the stress that brings on new outbreaks, and facts that should help allay unnecessary fears about herpesvirus. In Chapter 6 we'll examine some *good* ways to tell friends, family, and prospective lovers about herpesvirus—in a non-threatening, supportive manner—and hear from herpesvirus patients who have managed to cope successfully with this frustrating illness. But to be able to deal with herpes effectively, we first need a complete understanding of its nature and behavior.

2

The Anatomy of a Virus

Nature does nothing uselessly. — ARISTOTLE

What is a virus, exactly? In 1898, Dutch botanist Martinus Beijerinck discovered that certain diseases were caused by particles even smaller than bacteria. To describe them, he used the term *virus*—the Latin word for poison. The smallest known form of life, viruses can be seen only through an electron microscope. A micron, a unit of measurement developed only recently, is equal to 1/25,400 of an inch. A *large* herpesvirus is only one-third of a micron long!

As difficult as it may be to believe, scientists in the 20th century are still not able to state exactly what viruses are—nor are they able to say whether viruses are actually alive! Viruses exist in the twilight zone between living and non-living things. They do reproduce and evolve. But until they enter an acceptable host cell, virus particles simply do not behave like living organisms. In the introduction to his book on the subject, Dr. Wolfhard Weidle, a world-renowned expert in biochemical genetics, asks, "What is a virus?" And he answers himself:

> Let us admit at the outset that we do not know; there is no brief and precise definition of the term. Perhaps the only practical definition would be: "Virus is what we are going to talk about in this book."

In its study of these enigmatic particles, modern virology has been able to determine that all viruses consist of a *capsid*, or coating comprised of protein molecules, and a core made up of genetic material—either DNA (deoxyribonucleic acid), or RNA (ribonucleic acid), or both. These nucleic acids are complex molecules that exist in all plant and animal cells. DNA, usually found in a cell's nucleus, is the main substance of chromosomes—the stuff of heredity. When a cell divides, it produces two identical sets of chromosomes, so that the new cell's "daughter" is provided with complete genetic instructions for growth, reproduction, organization, and function. (Modern science has recently synthesized DNA molecules that actually divided—man-made structures that were, in a sense, alive.)

RNA is not restricted to the nucleus but can be found anywhere within a cell. It closely resembles DNA but has a somewhat different molecular structure and chemical base. Unlike DNA, it is essential for the development and production of all proteins.

The genetic instructions within the nucleic acids dictate replicative information, as well as other data, to plant and animal cells. But in order to reproduce, viruses require additional substances that they themselves do not possess. A virus, therefore, needs to find a live cell for the nutrients and other substances it needs to live and reproduce.

The shape of any particular virus is determined by the quantity and type of protein molecules making up its capsid. Herpesvirus particles, called virions, are usually sphere- or rod-shaped. This coating has a dual purpose—it creates a barrier that protects the viral RNA or DNA from potentially harmful substances in the host organism's environment, and it enables the virus to enter a host cell by attaching itself to a cell wall.

All viruses are parasitic—they can thrive only after they have entered the cell of a host organism, usually an unwitting one. It's been said that a chicken is merely an egg's way of making another egg. Similarily, it could be said that a cell is merely the method used by some viruses to further their own existence. To reproduce themselves, viruses invade cells and substitute their own nucleic acid for the genes within the invaded cell. By so doing, viruses "hijack" the host cell's genetic material and direct its metabolism in order to replicate themselves.

All forms of life, from one-celled organisms on up, are prone to viral infection. Viruses that seek out and invade bacteria are known as bacteriophages, or "bacteria eaters." Like higher forms of life, most bacteria have tough cell walls that are not readily penetrated. And so bacteriophage viruses have evolved a needle-like appendage. The virus pierces the bacterium's cell wall and then injects its genetic information, much as a doctor injects a drug into a patient via a hypodermic needle.

Viruses are a major cause of disease in plants and higher animals. Insects that feed on a plant's leaf and stem tear down walls of cellulose that would normally be too tough for a virus to penetrate, leaving open, damaged areas that permit viruses to enter. And insects themselves spread viral particles simply by moving from plant to plant. In turn, botanists help boost crop yields by infecting the local insect pest population with a crippling or fatal virus. And farmers have used a controversial technique—mass viral infections—to rid themselves of marauding rabbits.

Most viruses are strictly species-oriented. Rous Sarcoma Virus, for instance, is found only in chickens, but a few other viruses—such as rabies and anthrax—can be transferred from one mammalian species to another. But by nature, viruses become activated only in specific cells. Until a viral particle comes in contact with an appropriate host cell, it remains essentially inert.

For example, you may contract an intestinal virus by breathing air contaminated with the virus particles exhaled by an infected person. That virus's first contact with your system occurs in your respiratory tract. But even when breathed deep into your lungs, the virus particle remains docile—since it has not yet encountered any intestinal cells to invade. Ultimately, though, it will be absorbed from your lungs into the bloodstream and carried to the intestinal tract. There, in the presence of potential host cells, a biochemical reaction takes place. The viral proteins adhere to chemically-sensitive parts of the cell wall called *receptors*, and it's at this site that the virus inserts itself into the host cell. (In some of these interactions, only certain genetic information is passed into the cell, instead of an invasion by the entire virus.)

Once inside the cell, the viral DNA or RNA subverts the cell's own genetic instructions, causing it to duplicate proteins and nucleic acids to the virus's specifications. In effect, the virus overrules the cell. This abuse of the cell's natural function eventually cripples or kills it—but not before it has assisted the virus by reproducing viral particles in vast quantities. Inevitably, the cell wall bursts from the excesses of viral replication within, and the newly-created viruses disperse and encounter other healthy cells to invade.

Some of the more common human diseases caused by viruses include measles, influenza, the common cold, chicken pox, polio, shingles, encephalitis, hepatitis, mumps, smallpox, viral pneumonia, yellow fever and, of course, herpes simplex. Some of these viruses can exist within a host cell without damaging it; other viruses can cause cancer in both animals and plants. And within the past twenty years, new developments support the theory that viruses are factors in the development of cancer in humans (a subject discussed in greater depth in Chapter 9).

The Herpesviruses

Among viruses, the herpesvirus family is one of the most pervasive and resistant. Every animal species in existence is affected by at least one of the herpesvirus subgroups, which cause more disease in humans than any other virus.

The extremely common *Varicella–Zoster Virus* (or *VZV*) causes the childhood disease of chickenpox. Most people contract VZV in early childhood by breathing particles floating in the air, often at school where other infected children are present. (Prolonged exposure is usually required to contract VZV.) Only rarely are there complications with chickenpox, and full recovery is the norm.

But VZV later recurs in at least 80 percent of adults as herpes zoster. This virus is able to migrate into nerve pathways and lie dormant in the nerve ganglia. Later in life—particularly in elderly, or sickly patients—VZV particles become active again and retrace their original path to the skin surface, erupting into clusters of sores—an ailment known as shingles. Statistics suggest that most adults will eventually experience at least one shingles attack, sometimes as a result of some trauma to the area where the sores later appear.

Nerve pathways uniformly radiate into one side of the body or the other, and so the lesions of shingles generally restrict themselves to one side of the face, neck, back or extremities. For most shingle sufferers, the most troublesome problem is pain. Since most occurences of shingles occur in older patients, the sores can sometimes be quite slow to heal, and secondary bacterial infections of the lesions are not uncommon. Unlike herpes simplex virus, herpes zoster has an extremely low recurrence rate—less than five percent of those who suffer a shingles attack ever get a second infection. But herpes zoster is unquestionably contagious, and if an adult infected by shingles transmits the VZV virus to a child, the child will develop chickenpox.

Another common strain of herpes known as *Epstein–Barr Virus* (or *EBV*), causes infectious mononucleosis. In the United States, as many as 500,000 cases of the "kissing disease" (so called because it commonly occurs among adolescents making their first heterosexual contacts) are contracted each year, most in younger people between the ages of fifteen and thirty. Unlike VZV, EBV is very easily transmitted. As in herpes simplex infection, direct physical contact is required to get the virus. Some infected persons are contagious for many weeks before they even realize that they are carrying it.

Mononucleosis is known among clinicians as one of the "masquerading" illnesses. Initially, the infection makes a patient feel rundown and lethargic; and in its early stages, EBV is often misdiagnosed as leukemia, appendicitis, diptheria, hepatitis or strep throat. It often takes weeks—sometimes a full month or so—before "mono" becomes characterized by a high fever, muscle aches, chills, and more general fatigue. When the symptoms become debilitating enough to drive the patient to a doctor, blood tests can swiftly determine that the problem is mononucleosis.

Symptoms can last a full month and usually don't abate without severe sore throat, body rash, swollen lymph nodes, joint pain, and possibly even an enlargement of the spleen. Most people never develop symptoms but are known to have EBV antibodies in their bloodstream. Epidemiologists suggest that much of the population probably contracts EBV in childhood, but fights off the infection asymptomatically.

As with other members of the herpes family, there is no "cure" for a mononucleosis infection. No antibiotics are prescribed, but with adequate rest and good nutrition, the infection burns itself out in one to six weeks. Many patients jump the gun on their recovery, however, only to be rewarded with a relapse. (A relapse is not a recurrence; the disease has merely been weakened by the immune system but never fully conquered; and so is able to reinfect the body.) When patients exert themselves too soon, they use up more energy than the immune system can afford, allowing the virus to stage a comeback. But once the body rids itself of EBV, antibodies circulating in the bloodstream permanently prevent re-infection.

The least-known herpesvirus afflicting humans is *Cytomegalovirus* (or *CMV*), a dangerous and destructive infection. Oddly, random blood samplings of the population show that by age forty, almost 80 percent of all Americans have had some biological contact with CMV, as evidenced by the antibodies specific to that virus. CMV is spread only by direct contact, and causes illness only rarely in adults, in whom it manifests itself as a general viral infection (actually, a form of mononucleosis). An estimated 50,000 infants in the United States also contract CMV each year, but probably no more than 5,000 newborns actually develop the cytomegalic inclusion disease which causes blindness, hepatitis, mental retardation, enlarged liver and spleen, and nervous system damage. 5,000 out of 3.4 million live births is a tiny percentage, but a tragic one nonetheless.

An infant becomes susceptible to this wide range of serious disorders when its pregnant mother contracts CMV. The extent of CMV's toll upon the infant is determined by a number of factors, including the seriousness of the mother's infection and the virulence, or strength of the particular strain of herpes.

The last two members of this group, *Herpes simplex virus Type I (HSV–I)* and *Herpes simplex virus Type II (HSV–II)* cause most of the trouble discussed in this book.

These herpesviruses are spread only by actual physical contact. The virus particles are easily damaged by air, light, and temperatures significantly above or below 98.6°F, so it's rare for them to be spread via inanimate objects. In 1982, wire services all over the country ran a story about a young woman who alleged she used a lipstick sample in a Philadelphia department store and had severe oral herpes lesions break out in the exact pattern of the lipstick. Though it is possible that some contagious woman used the sample moments before she did, researchers have been unable to culture herpesvirus from lipsticks intentionally contaminated with viral particles. Another explanation is that the young woman may have been developing her own first oral herpes infection, and while using the lipstick sample, inadvertently spread her *own* virus around her lips.

To see precisely how the body reacts to an initial herpesvirus infection, let's trace the transfer of the oral form of the virus in a common mouth-to-mouth kiss.

A woman who has had recurrent herpesvirus infections is just getting over a cold sore that had appeared on her lip ten days before. Since childhood, her cold sores always occur at the same spot—at the right corner of her mouth. (Places where the skin folds or is stretched are favorite spots for herpesvirus to take hold.) Many people do not realize that cold sores are contagious at all, and this woman assumes that since the lesion is all healed except for the dry, crusty scab that is ready to fall off, her infection has passed the contagious stage.

Unfortunately for her boyfriend, she is wrong. Studies at research facilities throughout the United States and Europe have demonstrated that the virus can be cultured from the sites of lesions immediately *before* an impending herpesvirus infection is visible up until several days after the cold sore's last visible sign. (Virus particles have been cultured from the sites of lesions even after the scabs have fallen off.)

The young woman turns to her boyfriend and gives him a quick kiss on the lips. In that instant, she transfers one (or more) of the hundreds or thousands of viral particles.

From a virus's point of view, the corner of a man's lip is not a very congenial environment. The virion is exposed to drying, polluted air, at a temperature lower than the 98.6°F it is accustomed to. But by chance, it has come to rest on a cell on the surface of the mucous membrane. To avoid destruction, the herpesvirus' coat of protein molecules attaches itself to receptors on the surface of the cell.

Only certain viral proteins are able to attach themselves to certain receptors. Herpesvirus proteins, for example, can attach more readily to cells in the mucous membrane than to the tougher cells of the epidermal layers. But they can invade anywhere they get a chance to attach themselves to a cell. If people do contract herpesvirus through the skin, the virus usually takes hold through a cut or abrasion, where viral particles have access to less-resistant cells. (*Herpes gladiatorium*, usually caused by herpes simplex virus Type I, is commonly found on the elbows and knees of participants of close-contact sports, particularly wrestlers. The virions can enter the athletes' bodies anywhere the skin has been abraded or "mat burned." Like any other herpesvirus infection, this form will come and go, depending on many variables.)

It's possible to envision herpes simplex viruses as a group of terrorist hijackers. Terrorists usually have a goal to achieve and some idea of how to achieve it—but not the arms with which to achieve the goal. So what do terrorists do? They go out and commandeer a plane, causing international repercussions in the process. And so it is with herpesvirus. The particle's goal is replication. Within each virus's RNA and DNA is the "knowledge" of how to replicate. But because a virus has no mechanism for reproduction, the herpesvirus has to commandeer a cell and force it to produce new virus particles. Actually, herpesviruses are not malicious entities; they are simply programmed to replicate themselves as effectively as possible—and regrettably, they do a remarkably good job.

A cell's control center is its nucleus, which directs the cell's activity and carries out the instructions dictated by the genetic material within. Once inside the cell membrane, the virus particle—incredibly small, even on the scale of the cell—journeys to the cell nucleus and begins substituting its own genetic information. Its first "message" instructs the cell to stop all its normal functions. Having lost its self-determination, the cell follows the virus's next set of commands, which instructs it to replicate new herpesviruses—and at a very rapid pace.

The average cell taken over by a single viral invader can produce anywhere from 20,000 to 50,000 new herpesvirus particles a day—though the excess activity takes such a heavy toll that the cell won't live much longer than that. Soon the cell *lyses:* its exterior membrane deteriorates. New-formed viral particles spill out, and the cell dies. Countless herpesvirus particles, floating about in the cellular environment, affix themselves to other healthy cells nearby. The cycle repeats itself. Ever more cells begin lysing—spilling millions of virions, to infect still other cells.

At the same time, other viruses may be infecting cells without instructing them to produce more viruses. But unfortunately, these viruses are quietly incorporating their genetic data for future reference. Once the invaded cell has incorporated the virus's genetic information, it will manufacture a new set of "doctored" genes every time it divides. And such infected cells may then suddenly begin replicating virus particles.

Of course, the man in our example has not yet felt this subdermal cellular invasion. So far, the number of cells damaged is far too small. But slowly, a graveyard of what were once healthy, living cells begins to form. As each cell becomes overwhelmed by the subversion of its normal functions, the newly created viruses escape what's left of it and seek out new, healthy tissue to invade, using the captive cells' RNA to replicate still more viruses. The man is now able to feel irritation, burning, itching and tingling sensations at the site of the infection. The feelings caused by all of this microscopic activity is what doctors call the *prodrome*—sensations that are noticeable *before* a herpesvirus outbreak becomes visible.

Soon the area of the infection becomes swollen and inflamed. Tiny blisters form, filled with lymph fluid, dead and dying cells, virus particles, and white blood cells attracted by the trauma and commotion. At this point, the body's immune system must suceed in overpowering the viruses, together with the cells they have infected. Otherwise the viral rampage will continue, damaging so many cells that the entire organism may not survive.

3

The Immune System and the Problems of Recurrences

I couldn't imagine a worse experience. The pain in my groin was unbearable. I ran a high fever, had swollen glands, and unquenchable thirst and a throbbing headache. — CARRIE R.

Chances of surviving a viral infection depend on the virulence of the particular strain of invading virus, and the strength of the many different components of the host organism's immune system.

While a herpesvirus infection is underway, many different things are happening simultaneously. Immediately upon intrusion of a virus particle, the cell under attack begins to change. As its internal chemicals cease performing their normal functions, the molecular structure of its cell wall is modified by the presence to the virus within. Its biochemical coding changes, signalling to the immune system that the cell has been invaded.

Lymphocytes—one of the many types of white blood cells and one of the mainstays of the immune system—are always floating through the body, generally via the bloodstream and lymphatic systems. There are two different kinds: *T-lymphocytes*, known as T-cells, become warriors that go forth into the diseased areas. In the face of certain destruction, some of these T-cells will consume infected cells, often to die themselves from ingesting toxic substances.

B-lymphocytes, on the other hand, produce antibodies to fight specific invaders. When no trouble is evident, these "scouts" are relatively few in number. But when viral or bacterial invaders are discovered, these agents sound a biochemical alarm that stimulates the body to begin fast mass-production of other immune components. Spaced along the lymphatic vessels—like fuel and rest stops along superhighways—are lymph nodes. When people are ill with a viral or bacterial infection, they frequently develop "swollen glands"—actually engorged lymph nodes that have been spurred into action and are packed with lymphocytes.

In another form of bodily defense known as *cell-mediated* immunity, phagocytes and macrophages develop and scavenge the body in search of antigens to consume. *Phagocytes* ("cell–eaters") are the white blood cells that, like T-lymphocytes, consume infected cells and other foreign substances. Macrophages ("great eaters") are bigger cousins of the phagocytes. Although some macrophages and phagocytes are always circulating throughout the body, vast stores of them live and grow in the bone marrow, where they await the chance to defend the body in case of emergency. As these little defenders mature and die, others replace them, assuring the body a steady supply of "poison-eating" agents. Now, phagocytes and macrophages gather at the site of the viral infection, and begin enveloping and engulfing infected cells.

Other types of white blood cells contribute to the anti-viral attack. The B-cells, encountering a cell wall encoded with the chemical signals that indicate a herpesvirus invasion, will perform two functions. Some are stimulated to begin rapid division; others continue their circulation back to the lymph nodes, where their newly acquired chemical markings indicate that the body is under attack. The B-cells' molecular configuration can describe not only what sort of invader is responsible, but where the attack is taking place. The lymph nodes swell dramatically and step up their production of B-cells, which stream out of the lymph nodes and are carried to the site of the infection.

As the cellular graveyard on the lip receives more "corpses," the blisters swell and grow larger. Within days, they burst, and among the remains of the once-healthy cells are hundreds of thousands, if not millions, of extremely contagious virus particles. (A healthy respect for the fluid in these blisters can help limit the spread of herpesvirus—not only to other people, but to other locations on the sufferer's body.)

The sore on the man's lip is now quite noticeable and may be sensitive to the touch. With the immune system's heavy artillery in full operation, he may feel fatigued, achy, and low in energy. At the site of the infection, T-cells secrete toxins that attack viruses. They also motivate the "poison-eating" cells to work harder and remain at the site of the infection. Meanwhile, many B-cells are changing into plasma cells—which can concoct the proteins known as antibodies, which spread out over the surface of infected cells and code them, making them even more likely targets. In effect, the antibodies "scent" an infected cell and stimulate the macrophages to consume it, thereby halting further replication. Antibodies also interfere with the virus's ability to attach itself to cell-wall receptors.

To develop the proper antibodies, the body needs time—days and sometimes weeks (and in the case of newborn babies, several months). But in a primary herpesvirus infection, other components of immunity come into play. Many viruses cannot replicate themselves effectively in temperatures above 98.6° F —and thus a high fever can retard viral growth. The runny nose of the common cold also serves a purpose: viral particles by the hundreds of thousands are caught in mucous secretions, losing much of their ability to infect other cells elsewhere in the body.

Beyond merely signalling the presence of viruses within, an infected cell contributes to the defense of the body by secreting a substance known as interferon (see Chapter 13) for nearby, uninfected cells to absorb. While antibodies are designed to fight only specific invaders, interferon protects cells from a wide variety of different viruses and has even been shown to help resist the growth of certain cancers.

The immune system has numerous other defenses at its disposal, but too technical a discussion would only be confusing. The point is that in a relatively short time, all of them can come to the fore and effectively fight off a viral invasion. There is considerable variance, though—it will take anywhere from 12 hours to four days and in a primary attack, possibly longer—before this alliance of phagocytes, macrophages, T-cells, B-cells, plasma cells, antibodies, and interferon can turn the tide and get the viral attack under control.

This explains why the actual symptoms, extent, and duration of lesions vary widely from person to person. Some less fortunate individuals suffer chronic infectons. Somehow, the herpesvirus outnumber or resist the immune system and remain localized and active, with new lesions breaking out as old ones heal.

Although there has been no catataloging, some scientists believe that hundreds, even thousands, of separate herpesvirus strains exist. If so, then it's likely that some viruses are exceptionally weak and may cause only a mild, hardly noticeable primary attack. On the other hand, other strains may be particularly virulent. Patients who are subject to incessant, overlapping, never-quite-healing herpesvirus infections at the site of the initial outbreak may harbor a particularly strong strain of the virus—or have an unusually weak resistance (or, as is most likely, a combination of the two).

Typically, however, most lesions last from two days to two weeks, depending on the severity of the outbreak, the individual's general health, and site of the sore. When the blisters burst, the inflammation usually subsides. Within another day or two, the lesions begin to crust over, forming a scab that will last (again, depending upon a number of variables) for up to ten days. If the scab is continuously worn away by friction, scratching, or washing, then healing will take longer.

Scientific studies of the population indicate that most adults' blood samples show signs of antibodies lingering from past or present herpesvirus infections. By the age of fifty, between 75 percent and 90 percent of all American adults have herpes simplex virus (Types I or II) antibodies in their blood. About half of those affected by herpesvirus are never troubled again. But the other half will be subject to recurrent herpesvirus outbreaks that go through the same sequence of blister, sore, and scab—over and over again.

Why do these individuals suffer recurrences? Because unfortunately, herpes simplex virus has developed a behavior trait that allows it to survive in the face the body's valiant attempts to destroy it.

One of herpesvirus's unique (and most frustrating) qualities is its ability to retreat into a "safety zone" just as the body's natural defenses are gearing up to create a hostile, anti-viral environment. During the intercellular battle, some herpesvirus particles find their way into a nerve cell leading from the skin's surface. Somehow, these particles gain entry to the nerve axons—the pathways of the nervous system—and migrate along the neural pathways, or nerve paths, to the groups of nerve roots known as neural ganglia.

In vertebrates, the sensory ganglia are clumps of nerve cells located just outside the brain and near the base of the spinal cord. Like linking cables, these neurons transmit sensation from the skin to the brain. From the ganglia, neural projections reach in two directions. One "set" of nerves forms a pathway to the surface of the body in order to receive signals, and another pathway travels on from the ganglia to the brain, "advising," in a sense, what sensations have occurred.

Dr. Ernest Goodpasture's pioneering work with herpesvirus in animals has provided contemporary bioscientists with some excellent leads in studying the virus's unusual behavior. Dr. Goodpasture observed that "if the eye of a rabbit was infected with the virus, inflammations were seen along the nerves that convey sensation from the eye to the brain, and that the virus was found in groups of nerve cells [ganglia] near the brain and spinal cord; the nerve cells might be the sites where the virus set up permanent residence in the host. Over the succeeding years, studies . . . have demonstrated this to be true."

Dr. J. Richard Baringer of the Department of Neurology at the University of California at San Francisco and his staff have confirmed that viruses do indeed reside in the nerve cells during latency. Recent observations indicate that the virions migrate by moving across the Schwann cells that line the neural pathways from the skin surface to the ganglia. But researchers emphasize they have only *deduced* that this is what happens. No one knows definitely how—or why—the virus travels.

In oral (and facial) herpesvirus infections, the virions migrate to a cluster of nerve roots in the upper cheek, near each temple, known as the trigeminal ganglion. In the case of a genital herpesvirus infection, virions travel along the peripheral nerve cells to the lumbo-sacral ganglion, a cluster of nerve cells at the base of the spine.

Dr. Baringer has also studied how herpesviruses behave (or more exactly, fail to behave) while dormant. Though some viral replication may still be occurring at the site of the original infection, herpes simplex viruses that have found their way to the ganglia enter a latent, or dormant, state. Within nerve cells, herpesviruses don't replicate themselves. They simply exist there peaceably, remaining inactive until they "decide" to travel back along the neuron to cause a new outbreak at the site of the original infection.

Even though these virions within the neurons remain untouched, it's not the immune system's fault. Had the immune system failed, those virus particles would have replicated themselves millions of times, spreading lesions and swiftly consuming the entire body, until death occurred. But the immune system is designed to seek out and destroy *active* foreign bodies. In their inert state, the herpesviruses are completely harmless, so none of the body's many defense systems are motivated to hunt them down. And so, the inert herpes virions can remain there in the neural ganglion, unthreatening—and unthreatened.

Unlike most cells in the body, nerve cells do not reproduce. Once a neuron is injured or killed, it is not replaced. Hence, the human nervous system has evolved elaborate defenses. It is so self-protective that almost no bodies foreign to the nervous system can gain entry to the axons; even the immune system's antibodies are denied access. But perhaps because of their extremely minute size, herpesviruses *do* get in.

All forms of life seek nourishment, to protect themselves from their enemies and the harshness of their environment. Life forms that are able to adapt—by being stronger, faster, or more adept at hiding from enemies— will survive to reproduce. Earlier in their evolution, herpesviruses may have been larger than they are today; only the smallest of them were able to enter the highly-protected neural pathways and migrate to the sanctuary of the ganglia. If so, then only the very smallest herpesvirus particles survived to replicate themselves. Hence, generation after generation of natural selection ensured a succession of increasingly tiny viruses. But the sensitive nervous system continues to exclude any rambunctious antibodies that might go after an errant herpesvirus—and so this is how herpes can live on within the nerves without being eliminated.

Now and then, the virus will retrace the nerve pathway and return to the exact site of the original infection. Since there is no viral replication inside nerve cells, it is the *same* viral particles that make the trek back to the place where the new sores will develop. And in a sizable human being, the length of certain nerve pathways can be more than three feet long!

What stimulates latent viral particles to hike down the neural pathway to the original site of the infection and begin to replicate themselves? That's a question scientists have been puzzling over since the earliest investigations of herpesvirus. One school of thought holds that the herpesvirus is constantly monitoring the state of the body's immune system. The moment the body's defenses deteriorate for any reason at all, the viral particles launch an attack.

Another theory is that the virus lies dormant until the ganglion is stimulated (or overstimulated). This causes the virus particles to "get moving," over the original route they took after the primary infection. Again, this may be a survival trait developed over millions of years of evolution: when a host organism dies, the viruses in its body perish along with it. The herpesvirus particles may interpret stress or illness in their host as a possible sign of danger—and thus migrate back to the skin surface, where they can infect a new (and presumably healthier) host.

Back at that same area of skin, the virus particles begin to attach themselves to healthy cells and begin replicating. Only then, when the viruses have left the security of the nerve axons, can the immune system's antibodies come into play and wipe out the invading virons. But unfortunately, a few of the herpesvirus particles remain in the ganglion or nerve axon, and so survive the assault from the antibodies. It is herpesvirus's unique ability to rest quietly and unobtrusively that makes it such a successful parasite.

The Psychological
Dimension

4

Psychological Reactions

The greatest griefs are those we cause ourselves
— SOPHOCLES, *Oedipus Rex*

Sam Knox of the Herpes Resource Center says that, "For most people, herpes is not terribly debilitating, but it can be a horrible psychological problem." Dr. Fred Rapp agrees: "Even here at the research end I've observed that a big part of this problem is psychological. In most cases that I've seen, the lesions are not as severe a problem as one would think, having observed how upset the patient is. Unfortunately, many of these people feel that they are social outcasts."

When the National Genital Herpes Symposium was held in Philadelphia in 1981, Elliot Luby, M.D., Professor of Psychiatry at Wayne State University, delivered a presentation titled "Psychological Responses to Genital Herpes." Although Dr. Luby's remarks were directed mainly at health-care professionals, they also explored some of the less obvious psychological and emotional effects that accompany genital herpesvirus:

> Psychological factors are important in both the resistance to genital herpes and in the adaptation to the disease. The fact that it attacks young people during vital periods of psychosexual development makes it a pervasively crippling disorder in virtually all areas of living.
>
> The initial therapeutic contact is most often with the physician who diagnoses the disease. If the patient is treated abruptly or judgmentally, his anxiety and anger may be enormously heightened. Genital herpes is not a diagnosis that can be communicated with clinical detachment or insensitivity to emotional response.

Dr. Luby's point is borne out by the experience of Daniel K., a 28-year-old graduate student of engineering in Montreal. He contracted the virus five years ago when he was an undergraduate.

Daniel: *At first, when the doctor told me that what was causing my sore was genital herpes, I had little or no reaction. The woman I'd had sex with had kind of a wild reputation, and I was glad to hear that I didn't have syphilis or gonorrhea. But as I questioned the doctor more about the disease, I grew progressively more concerned. He was relaxed as we talked—patient, but almost distracted, like he saw it every day. Soon I learned that he had been seeing it every day—several times a day, as a matter of fact.*

But halfway through our conversation, I began to feel quite depressed. It was clear to me that the doctor was soft-pedaling the disease. There was no cure for it, and it stayed in the body indefinitely, recurring just about at will. He had nothing to gain by frightening me, but that was exactly what did scare me. If he'd said, "Look, this is a nasty problem, but it's not too serious," I might have felt a lot better. But I had the impression that he was keeping something from me. Maybe I've watched too many Marcus Welby's. I don't know. . . .

As Dr. Luby says:

There is a sequence of responses to genital herpes observed by clinicians and at herpes self-help centers:
1. Initial shock and emotional numbing which occurs as a reaction to any serious or life-compromising disease. . . .

Debbie R. is an administrative assistant in New Haven, Connecticut.

Debbie: *The crisis and the horror that you feel don't occur until you start to ask yourself those questions; until you learn more about the disease. Then it suddenly hits you that this goes away and comes back and goes away and comes back; and you don't really have much control over it.*

It didn't strike me traumatically all at once, as if I was suddenly told by a doctor that I had herpes. It was a slow-motion panic.

2. Following the shock, there is a frantic search for an immediate cure, or at least reassurance that the disease can be managed. . . .

Our society leads us to believe that nothing is really impossible—or at least, not for long. If we try hard enough, ask the right questions, see the right experts, we're bound to get an answer. But in terms of herpesvirus, that's not so. *Everyone* feels frustrated. The patients are frustrated; they can't get rid of it. The doctors are frustrated; they don't know how to cure it. Even the pharmaceutical companies are frustrated; they can't develop a wonder cure and make millions of dollars selling it. Eleanor C. Sloan, who received her degree in psychology from the University of Chicago, describes herself as an eclectic therapist and educational counselor. In her clinical practice in New York and Philadelphia, she explores the range of emotions that most herpesvirus patients experience. According to Mrs. Sloan, "People start to think, 'Someone out there has the answer, and they won't tell me.' Or, 'If only I had enough money, I could find the answer.' The frustration drives us to try gimmicks and fads." For many, herpesvirus is their first experience with an illness that won't go away in a week or two with the help of a doctor's prescription. And the feeling of not being in complete control—of not being able to pick up the phone and be cured overnight—is often devastating.

3.   As the shock subsides, there develops a sense of isolation and loneliness as awareness of the chronicity of the disease and its incurability breaks through the initial denial. Questions arise about the durability of heterosexual relationships, and patients experience a foreboding that life's dreams of companionship, sexual gratification, and children may not be possible.

Mrs. Sloan says that though oral herpesvirus may have been acquired through sexual contact, it does not seem to present the same debilitating emotional trauma. Why? Because, Mrs. Sloan speculates, American society of the 1980s may still be a bit more Victorian than the media would have us believe. If a virus breaks out on the lip, it's accepted as easily as a touch of the flu. But a sexually-transmitted disease carries a stigma.

Herpes Simplex Virus and Self-Image

Carrie A. drives a cab in Honolulu and first contracted herpesvirus one year ago.

Carrie: *I couldn't even be in pain in peace. I was scared to death of dying of a venereal disease. How would that look back in the local paper that my parents read? "Local Woman Dies of Mysterious Venereal Infection in Hawaii!"*

The high fever was making me delirious. I wasn't sure who gave me the infection, and in my delirium, I was struck with the urge to call every guy I'd slept with—not to mention a few women, too—and warn them they'd been with a disease-spreading nympho.

Long ago, Hippocrates stated: "It is more important to know what kind of person has the disease than what kind of disease the person has." For many of us, sex is deeply involved with our self-image. And when any disturbance unsettles our sexual behavior, it can play havoc with our self-image as well. It is most urgent for herpesvirus patients to absorb the concept that being subject to something is not the same as *being* that thing. One is *not* a herpes victim; but one *is* subject to occasional outbreaks of herpesvirus. Although a person may be subject to colds, poison ivy, and a cut finger (just as someone may be subject to herpesvirus), he or she *isn't* an affliction or a disease. Ill health is temporary, a passing condition. Herpes may be in the nerve ganglia to stay, but the recurrences are still temporary.

Always keep in mind that you are not a virus. Herpes, annoying and sometimes disruptive as it can be, is only a small part of who and what you are. As a whole *person*, you can reasonably expect that other people will relate to you, accept you, and sometimes reject you on the basis of the blend of elements and attributes that make you unique. Rarely will you be evaluated in terms of anything as one-dimensional as herpes, particularly if *you* don't see yourself that way. If someone tries to focus on this one element to the exclusion of all else, set him straight, or walk away—it's his problem, not yours.

4. As these concerns grow in intensity, anger becomes the dominant emotion—anger directed at the person who is the source of the infection can, in some patients, reach murderous proportions. It can also be focused on the physician, who is helpless to eradicate the disease and therefore disappoints the patient.

Whenever a herpesvirus recurrence breaks out, the patient is forcibly reminded of a sexual intimacy that took place weeks, months, or even years ago—with unpleasant results. Many times, the love relationship has long since broken up, and for most people, it's emotionally wearing to be constantly reminded of past unpleasantness.

George D., a 32-year-old math teacher from Omaha, contracted herpesvirus from his wife, who had been sleeping with other men without his knowledge. The disease brought into focus the basic problems in their marriage, which soon dissolved. But George still suffers outbreaks six to eight times yearly. Each recurrence forces him to reflect on the painful physical manisfestation of the disease, as well as the infidelity that led to his contracting herpesvirus in the first place. "Every time I get it, I cry and want to strangle her," George says. "I haven't seen her for five years, but I'm reminded of her all the time. It makes my blood boil."

Mrs. Sloan feels that rage, one of the emotions that she identifies in so many of her clients, can be exhausting—literally: "When we become enraged; when we get really angry, we don't see things so clearly. Rage is wearing. It distorts our judgment. It makes us isolated and insulated. Sometimes it makes us think, 'I'm a nasty person. I caught this terrible disease.' An illness like herpes can change an easy-going person into someone who's touchy, irritable, with a chip on the shoulder."

5. Fear generalizes to many areas of the patient's life. Anxieties about contagion, childbirth, and cervical cancer emerge. Women are understandably more affected by these fears than men. Should a potential lover be told about the herpes? What are the patient's obligations to tell anyone about the disease? Not only do women suffer more, but they feel a greater duty to tell.

Debbie R.: *I realized that I had a moral obligation to tell someone I was going to sleep with that I had herpes—whether or not I had an outbreak at the time. It brought on a whole new consciousness that was scary and upsetting to me—something that I have to deal with every time I meet someone I'd like to go to bed with.*

6. As time goes on, there is a "leper" effect. Patients describe convictions of ugliness, contamination, or even dangerousness. Some believe they deserve separation from the rest of society. Fear, shame, and guilt intensify social isolation because relationships require too much energy and become too complicated. There is a leper-like path to self-involvement, a retreat from intimacy and sexuality, and a move to a reclusive life. Many people become celibate, even religiously, moralistically anti-sexual.

During a recent lecture in Philadelphia, Mrs. Sloan pointed out that most people who suffer from genital herpesvirus infections are perfectly healthy in other ways. But because herpesvirus is transmitted sexually, those people stigmatize themselves and lose much of the perspective they once had about themselves.

Daniel K.: *For almost a year, I evaporated from the social scene. I didn't want to go out with anyone. I felt like a leper—literally. For a long time, until I learned more about it, I believed I would infect just about anyone with whom I went to bed. Tough on the ego, believe me! So I just withdrew and stopped dating—and I used to have a frantic social calendar.*

People noticed the change in me—it was obvious something was wrong. But I told no one. Of course, the two girls I had been seeing regularly thought that I had just lost interest in them, but it was really the herpes.

Debbie R.: *Emotionally, I was completely and thoroughly devastated. I never wanted to have sex again, and I pictured myself as an object of quarantine.*

According to Dr. Luby, this "leper" syndrome is accompanied by a morbid preoccupation with the disease:

These patients become obsessively involved with the adversary virus and the pain and discomfort it produces. Other interests gradually become less important as patients inspect their bodies . . .

Diane: *Do I think about herpes much? Yes, I guess. As a matter of fact, I think about it every time I go to the bathroom. I wonder if it'll hurt when I urinate. That's how the first attack began; I noticed it when I went to the bathroom.*

Take today, for instance: how many times did you think about herpesvirus infection?

[Diane laughs.] *Today at work I was so busy I didn't even have a chance to go to the bathroom!*

So you didn't think about herpesvirus at all?

[Laughing even harder:] *No! I didn't go to the bathroom, and I didn't think about herpes at all today.*

Some people become experts on the disease, as they explore the literature and eagerly await the results of new research. Unfortunately, this energy is committed at the expense of realistic adaptation to genital herpes, which would allow for a full range of living and continuing progression toward life goals and mature heterosexual relationships.

"Some people," observes Mrs. Sloan, "catch a cold, and two days later, it's gone. Other people catch a cold, and they still have a cold fourteen days later. Three *weeks* later, they're still complaining about it. In other words, some people get sick, and other people get *sick*. To them, a cold is really interesting; they can really get into it. They really *like* that cold, and having it is somehow necessary. It gives life meaning."

Similarly, people can often take up herpesvirus almost like a hobby, focusing all their attention on it. A 25-year-old nurse in Braintree, Massachusetts, has many friends, who like herself, have herpesvirus: "Some of them have lost their perspective about it. These people embrace herpes like a long-lost brother. It seems that if someone discovered a cure for herpesvirus tomorrow, some of these people wouldn't have anything to do. They'd have to readjust their whole lives. I don't ignore herpes or pretend that I don't have it, but I can't see waving the banner. It may be a pain in the ass, but really it's just a virus."

> 7. Depression deepens over time and with each recurrence. There are feelings of helplessness, hopelessness, unworthiness, guilt, self-hatred, and a deterioration in occupational performance. Some patients become suicidal as they feel a frustrating sense of entrapment. They believe that no one can help and that they are completely alone. Phrases like "If I had only done this or that," or "Why me?" are frequently uttered. Thoughts of this kind, of course, are often found in patients who have chronic diseases.

Mrs. Sloan agrees that a common—and powerful—response to genital herpesvirus is helplessness. "Sick people," she avers, "know they don't have to succeed. Sick people don't have to function. Being ill—with herpesvirus or anything else—provides an excuse, a rationalization for disappointment and isolation." Patients wallow in despair: "I can't get rid of it. There's nothing I can do." If left unresolved, feelings of helplessness can develop into feelings of hopelessness. Says Mrs. Sloan, "We tell the disease, 'Here I am, take me. I'm not worth much, because I've caught this nasty illness. So you take over; I'll give up.' "

Such an attitude sets the stage for not being able to cope—with herpesvirus, or any other illness. This attitude, in turn, creates a feeling of dependency. People come to depend upon doctors, other patients, even the predictability of the disease itself.

8. Finally, herpes may reactivate underlying psychopathology and

disorganize already inadequate coping strategies. Paranoid and conversion syndromes have been observed.

Some herpesvirus patients do cripple themselves psychologically by using their disease as an excuse to avoid interpersonal relationships—but that's a behavior pattern that they may have developed *before* herpesvirus came into their lives. Those who fail to adjust may become hermits, suffer debilitating depression anxiety, even contemplate suicide. But Dr. Luby is careful to point out that not all genital herpes patients are so affected. Happily, such extreme responses are rare—and most patients rapidly adapt to their recurrent infection.

"These patients," says Dr. Luby, "are generally older, married, and fully understand the disease. They have been open with their wives and husbands in the discussion of herpes and have sexual relations only during periods when there are no lesions." Still, Dr. Luby insists that physicians should become more sympathetic of herpesvirus patients:

> Time should be allotted for patient education and careful, concerned exploration of the patient's feeling about the disease. This should be done with a positive attitude that at least the disease can be managed, if not cured, at this time, and that a reasonably normal life, with all of the potential achievements and gratifications, is possible.

Karen B. is an 18-year-old waitress who dropped out of high school when she was 16, who lives with her parents in Sioux City, Iowa. Her experience shows the help a compassionate doctor can give.

> Karen: *Everyone in school always joked about VD, and when I first noticed the sores on my vagina, I was terrified. Here I was thinking I had syph or something. I was fifteen then. I cried all night long, but then I decided that I had better get it looked at by a doctor.*
>
> *I'm friendly with my aunt who understands things a lot better than my folks, and she arranged for me to see a doctor. I wouldn't go until he promised me over the phone that he would be confidential. He said that he wanted to help me, and that telling my folks wouldn't have anything to do with my health. He said if I wanted to tell my folks, that was between them and me.*
>
> *I went to see him with my aunt that afternoon, after school. He took one look and said, "You have a little virus infection." I was relieved, but then he told me some things about it that upset me—like it never goes away completely. And that if I ever get pregnant and have a baby, I'll have to tell the doctors so they can keep an eye on me because the herpes can kill an infant. . . .*

Some work out their problems for themselves. Others feel the need to confide in friends or relatives; others seek religious counseling or therapy. "Assessment of the patient's emotional state should be made at each visit,"

Dr. Luby states. "If the emotional distress is severe and adaptation does not seem to be proceeding, then referral should be made for either a herpes self-help center or individual psychotherapy . . . Referrals for psychotherapy should be considered if the infection pervasively disturbs and disorganizes a patient's life. Depression with sleep disorder, loss of appetite, or suicidal ideation should be referred to a psychiatrist. Any overt psychotic symptoms, such as hostile paranoid resolution of a patient's anxiety, should also result in psychiatric referral."

5

Seeking Psychological Help

---

*When you have faults, do not fear
to abandon them. —* CONFUCIUS

Daniel K.: *For me, most of the damage was in my head, not on my body. Before I had the problem with herpes, I never had given two seconds' thought to seeing a shrink. I thought that was for crazy people. But it took a crisis like this to open me up and make me receptive to something like therapy. To get out of my rut, I started to see a psychiatrist.*

Herbert R.: *Believe me, the reports associating herpes with cancer in women—that made me feel great! Now I was starting to think about the possibility of having killed women, really getting carried away with the guilt trip. I started to see a psychiatrist—other things were going just as badly for me. I wasn't losing it simply over the herpes, but that was the main problem. I saw myself as an alien—an infectious alien, at that.*

With the psychiatrist, I was able to get back into the frame of mind I was in before I let the disease get the better of me; back in the years when ignorance was bliss. The doctor helped me tremendously. Most of my personal progress was regarding the herpes thing, and the worst of my problems became the least. What I did was, simply, actually force myself back into the space I was in before I knew how dangerous herpes could be.

Why Psychotherapy?

Eleanor Sloan defines psychotherapy as the process of refocusing. Clinical psychotherapy is often defined as the use of psychological techniques to treat abnormal behaviors. But in either case, psychotherapy alters our perception of the world and ourselves to let us live more contentedly and productively.

Some therapies, such as psychoanalysis, can be strict and formal. Sigmund Freud (1856-1939) discovered that symptoms of hysteria would disappear when a patient discussed the symptoms while under hypnosis. Therefore, he theorized that personality disorders arose from the expression of painful and/or socially unacceptable thoughts and impulses. If people could become aware of their unconscious internal conflicts, they could resolve their emotional dilemmas. Psychoanalysis was Freud's technique for bringing repressed thoughts and feelings to consciousness. Usually the patient makes a significant investment of time and money, often having five therapy sessions a week for as long as five years—or more. The analyst presents insights into the patient's behavior, using such techniques as free association of ideas and interpretation of dreams.

Client-centered therapy is based on the methods of psychotherapist Carl Rogers. Rogerian therapy uses verbal exchange as the means of influencing the patient's behavior. In his book *On Becoming a Person*, Rogers expresses his belief that humans are basically "positive in nature . . . basically socialized, forward-moving, rational, and realistic." Client-centered therapy establishes an environment of warmth, trust, and acceptance that permits the patient to express repressed subconscious thoughts without fear of the chastisement or disapproval that society generally offers.

Both psychoanalysis and client-centered therapy are subject to the criticism that simple awareness of internal conflict is not necessarily sufficient to alter behavior. Behavioral therapists seek active changes in their patients. They believe that behavior disorders are learned and can therefore be modified or eliminated. The three stages of behavior therapy are *extinction, reinforcement*, and *shaping*. Some varieties of behavioral therapy include aversion therapy (negative reinforcement), desensitization (conditioning to reduce phobias) and observation (in which patients who fear dogs, for example, observe others handling puppies without harm).

For those who want to explore the various possibilities, *The Complete Guide to Therapy: From Psychoanalysis to Behavior Modification* by Joel Kovel, M.D. (Pantheon Books, 1976) is encyclopedic in its detailed accounts of traditional and innovative therapies available. Especially useful is the section entitled "A Guide for the Perplexed"—a question-and-answer discussion of the hows and whys of therapy. For treatment rendered by a psychiatrist or psychotherapist, some health plans provide different schedules of reimbursement, depending on whether the therapist is an M.D. Before embarking on a course of therapy, you should make an inquiry to the health plan's administrator.

The therapies outlined above—including casual and relaxed exchanges such as talking it out with a bartender or cab driver—are traditionally one-on-one. In group therapy, patients sharing similar problems or experiences are brought together to benefit from personal interaction and the mutuality of experience. In September of 1979, the Herpes Resource Center saw an opportunity to provide just this service to herpesvirus patients. "It became obvious," says Sam Knox, "that some members needed a more direct, traditional self-help approach to develop coping strategies. We needed to help people get together—people at various stages of adaptive or maladaptive development who shared a common concern—to discuss their problems in a constructive atmosphere. We developed these chapter services for people who *have* worked out ways to cope and for those who haven't. It caught on like wildfire. There are now some fifty chapters nationwide."

> Daniel K.: *Another thing that helped me tremendously was to join a support group of people who all had herpes. I was shocked to hear my exact words and thoughts being spoken by other people. The experience of learning to deal with herpes is different for everybody, yet it is so much the same it's amazing. We talked about our feelings and our experiences. It was through the group that I decided to start going out again. . . .*

During her primary infection, Carrie E. stayed in her apartment, nursed by friends for the three weeks it took her to get back on her feet: "Some friends set up an informal around-the-clock nursing arrangement for me. In a little less than a month, I was completely recovered—physically." That's when she went to a HELP support group meeting at the local university and credits it with having "saved my life, emotionally."

> Carrie E.: *Right after I came down with herpes, I had so many confused and angry feelings I didn't know where to start to feel. The support groups have been really important for me therapeutically. Slowly, I sorted everything out. Through the support group, I learned to stop resisting my feelings. They're there for a reason—just as physical pain exists to warn us that something is wrong. Feelings—good and bad, happy and sad—all exist for a reason. It helps to get things out of your system, and to see that others are going through the same things.*

Tom R., a 35-year-old claims adjuster from St. Paul, is recently divorced. The complications of herpesvirus greatly compounded his anxiety over re-entering the world of dating. He first attended a HELP-sponsored support group after hearing about it from a friend who also had herpesvirus.

> Tom: *Although I already suspected that I had herpes, after I was diagnosed I went into a deep depression for a few days. But then the smoke started to clear. A friend at work had it, so I wasn't embarrassed to tell him about it. He told me about the support groups and invited me to one they were having—thank God!—that weekend.*
>
> *Any nervousness I felt, anticipating a room full of diseased sex freaks, vanished as soon as I got there. Everyone was understanding. Everyone seemed normal and conversant. I wasn't alone, and I didn't have to go into hiding or give up sex forever. That was a great relief. I had been told these things before, but the meeting was like a TV docu-*

mentary, live and before my eyes. I didn't say much, but I left that room a much different person, and immensely better off.

There should be a law that anybody who gets herpes should attend at least one support group meeting. It really does take the sting out of herpes, because for most people the worst part is the psychological oppression that comes with the territory. The support groups help relieve that burden.

Carrie E.: *The support group meeting gave me more than I can describe. Hearing those people at the support group—well, that turned my world around. I learned that some twenty-five million Americans have herpes, and maybe more than a hundred million worldwide. That diminished my feeling of being alone in a war of microbes. With the help of the group's leaders and the other people, I came to understand the most important thing—that this disease is really nothing more than an annoying, obnoxious virus.*

Sometimes I'm amazed at how open we can be in the support meetings. It's probably because we realize that we're all in the same boat. Even the criticism is more like pointed questioning. You can see people struggling with their own dilemmas in the questions and comments they raise. In part, that's what we're there for, to talk it out.

Of the herpes self-help groups (including those initiated by the American Social Health Association), Dr. Luby has this to say:

One assumption of these groups is that only people with the same problem or disease can understand and help each other. Another assumption is that people who help the most receive the most help. Herpes self-help groups attempt to work with newly diagnosed patients to achieve several goals:

•   *Ventilate rage.* The anger of a person with genital herpes can be disruptive. The self-help groups provide a forum for this anger, probably forestalling any serious acting-out. Yet this rage can be enduring, and its repeated expressions may not relieve it.

•   *Relieve isolation and loneliness.* The realization that others have the "dread disease" and are somehow managing is very reassuring. Observing that the "veterans" are composed, free of depression, and actively confronting life restores hope.

•   *Establish a new social network.* Many people give up old relationships because of shame, guilt, and fear of revealing herpes. It is comforting to be with others where there is no need to explain, no fear of rejection.

•   *Provide behavioral models.* For the herpes novitiates, mentors can be found among the "veterans." So often the new patients believe that no one else has ever suffered in the same manner. Sharing feelings and fears with others who immediately and empathetically understand appreciably reduces anxiety.

Appendix A includes a full listing of herpesvirus counselling and discussion chapters in cities around the United States, sponsored by the

Herpes Resource Center, whose services undoubtedly provide the best emotional support for those troubled by herpesvirus.

The Herpes Resource Center

The American Social Health Organization, a non-profit group, has been helping to solve the problems of sexually-transmitted diseases for 73 years. Most of ASHA's programs are targeted to bacterial diseases such as syphilis and gonorrhea, which, unlike herpesvirus infections, are curable. In May of 1979, ASHA created HELP, a national herpesvirus information program. Now known as the Herpes Resource Center, it boasts more than 30,000 members and is still growing.

Sam Knox, a graduate of New York University who worked for six years in the VD control program at Atlanta's Centers for Disease Control, is ASHA's National Program Director. Knox was the original architect of the Herpes Resource Center and says he is "delighted with HRC's performance because it's getting at a large number of people who need our services."

Has the media been responsible for the recent burst of attention given to herpesvirus?

Sam Knox: No question about it, herpes is over-hyped by the media. Even the usually most responsible outlets can't seem to resist exploiting the issue, and a lot of reporting is inaccurate and incomplete. But at least the media brought herpes into the public eye.

The press reports that there are some 20 to 40 million cases of genital herpesvirus in the United States.

I think forty million cases is high. Remember, not everyone who has genital herpesvirus is troubled by it. Some cases never recur. And many people are in relationships—marriage and otherwise—in which one or both partners have it, and are highly supportive of each other; and where herpes is not problematic.

What about the incidence of new cases?

The statistics most commonly heard—and they are probably accurate—are that half a million or more new cases of genital herpes develop every year.

For most sexually-transmitted bacterial diseases, intervention leads to successful treatment and cure. We have the national VD Hotline, a toll-free number to help people get medical treatment. We perform crisis intervention. People who are frightened; young people worried about their parents finding out. And the educational material we distribute has the same goal: to help people understand their problems and remove them from the infectious reservoir and into medical treatment.* But herpes—a viral, not a bacterial infection—is different. It can't be cured. That's what led to the establishment of the HRC.

Your organization used to be called HELP. Was that an acronym?

No, although we heard many guesses as to what it stood for. But we needed a name that would directly relate the program to the service—and in late 1981, we changed the name to the Herpes Resource Center.

What is the purpose of the Herpes Resource Center?

To help people, to increase awareness about herpes, and to enable patients to cope with the disease.

The HRC attracted a large membership quite quickly. Apparently it filled a need.

It did then, and it fills the same need now. The HRC was expanded to include other services, such as a special hotline for members. It's not toll-free. The number is given only to members and it's staffed by a health educator we employ, who can answer the immediate compelling questions raised by people who have herpes and have to have quick answers. The health educator has access to the very latest herpes information, and is experienced with lots of phone calls. All those insights can be shared with people on an immediate feedback basis to clarify uncertainty.

What is the main point about herpesvirus that the HRC is trying to communicate?

The basic premise is, once you have herpes, you have it forever. There is no cure, and basically, no treatment, either. It will recur periodically, people will be infectious periodically, and it's particularly important that the herpes patient know about potential consequences. This requires that we educate people who have herpes about self-care and personal hygiene, prevention, and the appropriate responses once you have the disease. That's what the HRC was trying to do when it was first structured and it's pretty much what it remains today.

Three years after its inception, the HRC furnishes its members four basic services: *The Helper* newsletter, the chapter services, the private hotline, and the organization of national symposia—which are not restricted to members. In fact, the symposia aren't directed primarily to our membership base at all; though members are, of course, welcome and many attend. The symposia serve to educate the public, and the cost is nominal. We bring notable experts in the field to discuss—in lay terms, to a predominantly lay audience—some of the complex medical issues that one would otherwise have to spend years in the medical libraries to ferret out.

---

* Those with questions about sexually-transmitted diseases other than herpes should call the toll-free National V.D. Hotline:
  (800) 227-8922 (for any state except California)
  (800) 982-5883 (for California residents only)

THE PSYCHOLOGICAL DIMENSION

What do you want the HRC's various services to do for herpesvirus patients?

They should come away with an understanding that, "I have this chronic condition called herpes. I am not a herpetic; I am not the virus itself. I just have this thing that requires some attention and care, but little more than that. Herpes doesn't restrict my life or preclude my enjoyment. It doesn't mean that I can't get married, have children, or be as fulfilled as anyone else."

What's the most important service the HRC performs?

All of our services are important, but the primary one is our quarterly newsletter, *The Helper*. Open and frank discussion about the problems and consequences—emotional as well as physical—of herpes, how to cope with it, how to deal with it in a basically single and sexual society; its unique problems in marital situations. Most importantly, *The Helper* furnishes a sense of hope: that herpes is not being ignored; that there is investigation and inquiry; that there's a tremendous amount of interest and research into the whole issue. The newsletter provides herpes patients with things they really need.

Another major reason for *The Helper's* development is that with the media giving herpes so much attention, reporting often accents the sensational and the bizarre, rather than giving a complete, authoritative, and balanced view of the facts. We wanted to give an alternative to sensational reporting on the issue. When the question of cancer comes up, as it inevitably does, popular publications deal with it in only partial detail. In *The Helper*, we can give full balanced coverage. In knowing more about herpes, one learns that it's not quite as threatening as originally portrayed in the popular press. And therein lies the program. Though we are nonprofit, our basic "product" is *The Helper*—which, by the way, was greatly expanded in form shortly after we published the first issue in May, 1979.

Over the years, The Helper *has printed increasingly detailed technical information. Do you think that might confuse some of your readers?*

Absolutely not. *The Helper* isn't too technical at all. Though we do print some technical material, we do so to provide the substantive detail that some of our members seem to want. It's a direct result of the membership's desires. They've expressed an interest in more information, in more detail than they're getting in the lay press. They want and need to be kept informed and able to make their own determinations.

People interested in learning more about herpesvirus and the Herpes Resource Center or those wishing to subscribe to *The Helper*, should send a stamped, self-addressed envelope to: Herpes Resource Center, P.O. Box 100, Palo Alto, CA 94302.

In addition to organizing support groups and counselling herpesvirus patients, some local HELP chapters publish their own regular or sporadic newsletters which advise members of local meetings, lectures, support group schedules, and medical news. One of the best we've seen is called *The Outbreak: A Recurrent Newsletter*, written and distributed by HELP/Philadelphia. *The Outbreak* takes an original and light approach to its serious subject. Some issues contain comic strips depicting herpesvirus-related plights. One year-end issue began with the words "Lesions Greetings," and another headline paraphrased comedian Henny Youngman: "Take My Herpes—Please."

6

Discussing Herpesvirus with Others

But in the year or two, herpes has been getting a lot of press. Everywhere I go it's herpes, herpes, herpes. — HERBERT R.

Question: Why do some people say they'd rather get syphilis than herpesvirus?

Clearly, it's best not to contract *any* disease, sexually transmitted or not. People who say they'd prefer syphilis to herpes simplex virus are probably referring to the fact that syphilis is curable. Although an individual can contract syphilis again and again, it is not recurrent: repeated bouts are the result of recontracting the spirochete. Herpesvirus, on the other hand, is incurable.

Making new friends and lovers (and keeping old ones) is hard enough as it is. For most herpesvirus patients, one of the most trying experiences is informing a possible sex partner about the dynamics of the disease—especially since the media has focused on the most dramatic and frightening aspects of genital herpesvirus.

After *Rolling Stone* published a pair of features on the subject, one reader wrote that the articles "did more for birth control than the Pill ever could. They made me almost not want to have sex." Kiki Olson, a writer for Philadelphia's weekly *Welcomat*, recently devoted a column to the herpes problem:

> My brother is an effortlessly attractive, personable 22-year-old. Like most budding boulevardiers, he frequents singles bars that feature a youngish crowd, extended happy hours and bargain-priced beers. But he can no longer be unconcerned about sexual experimentation.
>
> The Herpes Scare isn't just putting-off American college seniors from sexual forays. Last month, when I was in France, middle-aged Parisian businessmen were mentioning that they've cut down their on-the-road dalliances for fear of bringing something back to the 16th Arrondissement.
>
> As the epidemic continues, more people are bound to start

wondering "Does she?" "Suppose he?" . . . and come to the conclusion, "Hell, it's not worth it."

In this chapter, we'll explore—through personal interviews—how some individuals afflicted with herpesvirus related their dilemma to friends and potential lovers. Everyone seems to have his or her own approach. At one extreme, some individuals choose to ignore their malady and proceed without giving their sexual intimates the opportunity to make their own decisions about taking the chance of catching the virus.

> Karen B.: *Who'd go to bed with me if they thought they'd get herpes? Look, I don't want to give it to anyone else, but I don't want to ruin my whole sex life either. I love sex. If I'm having an infection, I just don't have sex. I'm pretty careful; I don't think I've given it to anyone else, and I hope I never do. But I couldn't bring myself to actually tell anyone about it—with one exception. If ever I find someone who I'd like to marry, then of course that would be different. But just guys I go out with? No way.*

> Carrie R.: *Several times, one woman has brought guys she wanted to sleep with to the support group meetings. She insisted that her lovers be fully aware of what they might be in for, in case anything was to go wrong and they caught it. Personally, I thought she was just absolving herself of any guilt in advance. But I'm not in a position to judge. Sometimes I go to bed with a guy without telling him about it—but only when I know I'm not having an active infection.*
>
> *Some people at the group criticize that attitude. One guy objected and said that he had herpes because a women didn't think she was contagious, but she was. He felt he should have had the opportunity to make a choice for himself. But he never had that chance, and now he has something else—herpes.*
>
> *I see his point. I'm not obstinate, but everyone has to make his or her own decision. I do it my way. Sometimes it's not worth the emotional pressure that's required to tell someone about it.*

This what-they-don't-know-won't-hurt-them attitude is especially common when an individual is just learning to live with the disease. Debbie R. caught herpes from her laid-back boyfriend—and picked up his casual attitude as well:

I was in an exclusive relationship. He didn't know he had it—or so he claimed. He pointed out a blister to me and said that it hurt him; that he'd gone to a doctor about it, and the doctor said it was nothing. Being totally ignorant about herpes or veneral disease, I really didn't even think about it. Later, I learned that he gets an outbreak every two or three years. I don't think he really knew what it was.

I didn't realize the full implication of having herpes. I was seeing only him, so it didn't occur to me that I might have to deal with this disease in terms of other men. Before our relationship was over, officially, I did have sex with someone else—and I didn't mention herpes to this other person. It seemed to be an absolutely safe one-night-stand situation, and I felt that I was safe herpes-wise, so I didn't think I should have to tell him about it.

The crisis developed when my boyfriend and I parted company. Suddenly, I was faced with having herpes and not having a comfortable sexual outlet. But I was able to do this amazing denial. I didn't bother to ask myself too many questions because I was in school, I was working, and not sure of where I was going. I allowed myself to be in a sort of limbo. I didn't even try to find out about the disease or look for information.

Later, I met this guy who I had known—through friends—for a long time. Once we got together and slept together, and I didn't tell him about it either. At the time, I knew I wasn't infectious. But I ran away from that relationship, partly because of the herpes, and partly for other reasons. For one thing, he was quite a lot younger than me.

Then I came in contact with a local HELP group, and attended a lecture at the university. It was horrible! At the lecture, I was really upset because I was learning all these terrible things about the disease. Up until that point, it was just something that was at the back of my mind, and I didn't have to think about it. There was an air of seriousness that frightened me. That night was the worst that I've ever felt about herpes. In looking back, though, that experience was something that had to happen. I needed it to wake me up.

Have you ever told anyone that you have herpes after having been in bed with him?

Yes, and believe me, I suffered through that! The anxiety building up to actually telling was terrible.

How did you tell him?

I just called him up the next day and said, "Listen there's something I should have told you last night, but didn't, so I'm telling you now. . . ." I told him calmly, and he simply asked, "So what?" He didn't care. Maybe he had it himself!

Have you ever told anyone about it who then refused to have sex with you?

Yes—the first man I ever told. Beginner's luck! He'd been a friend of mine for a while, and he had a lover. He claimed that he wasn't concerned about himself, as much as he was worried about bringing herpes into the other relationship he was engaged in.

How'd you take that?

I cried and screamed and kicked. It was a mess, but I was lucky—I guess. He stayed the night, and held me and tried to comfort me. It wasn't a rejection of *me* as much as a rejection of having sex with me. Looking back, it was pretty nice, and oddly, it made us better friends.

Finding a comfortable way to tell a prospective sex partner about herpes simplex virus can easily be the most dramatic chore in the life of an average herpesvirus patient. But it's not impossible. The more the general population learns about herpesvirus, the less frightening it becomes. And surprisingly enough, most herpesvirus patients report positive experiences when discussing their problem with others. Believe it or not, there are actually some personal *benefits* to telling others about herpesvirus.

Jacqueline T. is a secretary who works in San Francisco:

Have you ever told someone you might actually like about your herpes?

Yes. It must have been about five or ten people. The most successful time, though, was the most recent one.

What do you mean by "successful"?

I mean I came away from the conversation feeling pretty good about what I said and pretty good about how the other person responded. The sexual outcome is not the point.

What was the setting of this conversation?

Well, this man is an instructor of mine, and one day after class we were sitting alone, having a cup of coffee and talking about nothing in particular. We seemed to have a mutual attraction. I picked a point in our casual conversation completely irrelevant to herpes and told him about HELP. After that point, I knew he'd be wondering whether I had herpes. I wanted to get that out of the way, way up front in our relationship.

Were you planning to tell him about it?

No, but suddenly the opportunity presented itself, and I took it. There's this moment when you admit—I can't really describe it. I haven't done it *that* much, but it's kind of a confession. You wait for the ceiling to cave in, for your mother to walk through the door at the crucial moment. You wait for the person you're telling to faint or throw up. You wait for all those ridiculous things that never happen. Then to cover up that anxiety, I talk about things at a rapid pace: "It's not really so bad, and I've learned to cope by blah, blah, blah. . . . " You launch right into this pattern, just to talk, really.

What was his immediate reaction to your telling him that you had herpesvirus?

He wasn't embarrassed about it at all. He said, "Oh, that must be painful for you," in a consoling, not patronizing way. It's such a relief that the terrible reaction you expect never materialized.

It's not the conversation itself that I found so successful, but the whole *experience*. I really felt good afterwards, and I could see that he was still interested in me. The idea of going to bed with someone who has herpes wasn't scaring him off—now it was really out of the way, and that I'd discussed it as openly and as honestly as I knew how. I was as clear as I could have been with anybody. It was the right way for me to have that conversation.

Then our romance picked up with a great intensity. We didn't discuss herpes very much more for some time. Then he wanted to know what his chances of getting it were. I told him I couldn't give him a hundred-percent guarantee of *not* getting it, but I gave him my word that unless I was absolutely certain that I wasn't having an outbreak, that I wouldn't have sex with him, and that I'd do everything possible to prevent him from getting it. I promised that I wouldn't knowingly put him at risk. I said I knew he had to give it some thought, because having sex with me *is* a risk, period. I gave him my best estimation of what the risk was, and said I wouldn't jeopardize him. That was all I could do.

What was his reaction?

He said "Fine," and that he really wanted to hear me say those words. The best part was that we had the luxury of lots of time to discuss it before jumping into bed. I think that because we had so much time, things worked out perfectly. One of the most difficult parts about telling others about herpes is that often you don't have lots of time. People generally want to get into bed right away.

"How, Where, When, and What to Tell a Sex Partner About Genital Herpes," an article that appeared in the June 1980 (Vol. II, No. 2) issue of *The Helper* has several important cautions ("never use the word *incurable*") and some useful guidelines ("Assume that the person you are about to tell . . . knows nothing about the infection"). We reprint it here in slightly condensed form:

> When telling a sex partner about herpes, honesty and openness are the best policies from every point of view—ethically, humanistically, and even legally. Often unresolved, however, are the myriad strategic and tactical problems of *how* to tell, *where* to tell, and *what* to tell—in short, the tough stuff.
>
> To create some order in this otherwise murky and uncharted stretch of experience, HELP conducted a series of in-depth interviews and convened several discussion groups composed of the world's greatest experts on the subject—you. Those whose insights helped make this possible insisted—and rightly so—that this report not be couched in heavy, somber, or melodramatic terms. The underlying problem is heavy enough without adding to it. Therefore we decided to opt for a light treatment of what, without humor, might be an unbearable burden. The following report represents the collective wisdom of over two dozen people who, in the aggregate, account for more than 173

person-years of herpes and over eighty-five personal success stories, "almosts," and what could only be termed disasters, near-misses (and misters!), and strange encounters of every conceivable kind.

Before getting to the Dos and Don'ts, a few Nevers might be worth getting out on the table:

• *Never* use the word *incurable* when explaining herpes to another person. Not only does this word have unfortunate connotations and imagery attached to it, but it's inaccurate. Herpes is *very* curable—in fact, your body cures you again and again each time a recurrence goes away. Unfortunately, the virus has the ability to "hide out" and escape the otherwise lethal effect of your immune system; and therefore, the potential for recurrences exists. A better way to describe what's going on might be to refer to herpes as an intermittent, self-limiting condition that comes and goes more or less on its own, isn't particularly dangerous, and can be dealt with by the body, unassisted by drugs of any sort. That sounds better—and is more accurate.

• *Never* preface your remarks to another person with anything that sounds even remotely like, "I've got this terrible thing to tell you about myself," or "Better sit down, I've got this real heavy thing to lay on you." Your attitude makes a big difference!

• *Never* tell an untruth about herpes. Stick with the facts as you know them. Remember, you risk your credibility and compromise your ability to be a helpful source of information to another person if you allow even one white lie to slip in.

The Dos and Don'ts

• *Do* assume the person you are about to tell about herpes knows nothing about the infection. You will be right much more often than you'll be wrong. And even if the person knows something, chances are that what he or she knows is factually inaccurate or laden with inappropriate images.

• *Do* open up the subject at any convenient time. The consensus of our panel of experts was that there is no "right" time, place, or setting. Any time is the right time as long as you can talk without undue interruption and at length, so that as questions arise, they can be handled expeditiously and in detail. However, a number of times, places and settings were considered particularly inappropriate—at a crowded party where the noise level is such that you must shout to be heard; while having dinner for the first time at his or her parents' home; or having made love for the sixteenth time.

• *Do* follow your own sense of what is right in deciding when to bring up the subject. If you would have liked to have learned about herpes before having become infected, use this as a guide in making your choice. The overwhelming opinion was that people have the right to know what they're getting into *before* they're in the midst of it.

- *Do* use unprejudiced and generally neutral terminology in explaining what herpes is, what it does, and what it's like to have it. Also, try to start simply, and lay a solid foundation before launching into the complex molecular biologic aspects of the disease. For instance, a good way to begin is by asking the other person if he or she knows what a cold sore is (almost everyone does) and using that neutral analogous condition as a springboard into a discussion of genital HSV. One of the worst, generally *least* helpful things you can do is start throwing around words and terms like "DNA," "RNA," "replication," "caspid," and "genome" before you have explained herpesvirus.

- *Do* use whatever resources you have at your disposal to make your job easier or the understanding of the other person more complete. For example, don't hesitate to ask a knowledgable friend or doctor to help you explain what herpes is. Certainly don't hesitate to use HELP materials, past issues of *The Helper*, or even the Helpline to get answers to your questions or those of the person you are trying to tell.

- *Do* be sensitive to the reactions of the person you are telling, and be constantly reminded that how your express yourself, your choice of words, and even your body posture have some bearing on the outcome of your tête-à-tête. You simply may not have realized it before, but you do influence how other people will react upon learning that you have herpes.

- *Don't* use words like "nightmare," "malignant," "herpetic," "lesion," or "venereal" or any other words that are vague, subjective, scary-sounding or just basically obnoxious. If you think a word might be worth dumping, dump it—your instincts are probably right, and there are few words for which better substitutes don't exist.

- *Don't* worry in advance about telling. It doesn't help.

- *Don't* feel as though you have to be a walking encyclopedia about herpes. Tell it as you know it, and should questions come up that you could use some help answering, that's one of the services that HELP would be honored to provide.

- *Don't* forget to emphasize how preventable herpes is, particularly when people are informed, motivated, and sincerely eager not to spread the infection. Ditto insofar as the potential problems with babies, cervical cell changes and self-spreading to other parts of the body are concerned. All are easily prevented and/or dealt with to the point where risks are low. An important *Do:* If you are going to mention infectiousness, mention the other side of the same coin—preventability. If you are going to talk about elevated cervical cancer risks, also mention that the PAP test may be the saving grace. Make a point of being balanced in thinking and speaking about HSV. Let's not focus on so narrow a slice of the entire issue that we distort it.

- *Don't* be surprised if the person you are anxious about telling also has herpes and has been anxious about telling you. With the prevalence of genital herpes estimated to be in the millions, there's more than a remote possibility that one-quarter to one-third of all the new people you meet have genital herpes.

One of the men we interviewed agrees with this last point:

Herbert R.: *I have several women-friends who I see more or less regular-ly. They all know about my herpes, and it doesn't bother them—I guess because they trust me and know how careful I am about watching out for it. One of them later confessed to me that she'd had herpes on and off for years. She even reminded me of a date that she'd broken last summer, saying that she had caught a virus. Of course, she wanted me to think that it was a regular virus. But actually she had a recurrence and didn't want to go out and then refuse to have sex.*

We just laughed about it. Now, you see, I have a completely dif-ferent perspective about herpes. But the whole process of learning about it, understanding it, and finally coming to grips with it took me fifteen years. For me, it was a matter of attitude.

The reason for telling others about herpesvirus in the first place is so that your prospective sex partners can make a rational decision about pro-ceeding with physical intimacy. Therefore, it's vital that you present the in-formation in a clear, unemotional way. Eliminating the word "herpes" might be a good place to start. Whispering "I have herpes" in a hushed tone usually frightens and confuses people. And since the word "herpes" isn't fully descriptive, it can pose more questions than it answers.

The word itself sounds threatening and, in and of itself, it's in-complete. *Herpes* is a prefix for other terms: herpes simplex virus, herpetic eye infection, herpes simplex encephalitis, neonatal herpes infection, *herpes labialis*. What causes the most common grief and anxiety is the herpesvirus sores that appear genitally—*herpes progenitalis*. So let's refer to this virus accurately by using the term *herpesvirus*. It helps others understand what this malady really is, and more importantly, reinforces your own concep-tion of the disease. If you anxiously tell another person, "I have herpes," it sounds pretty serious. But if you say, "Every now and then, I have a bout of herpesvirus," it sounds more like an admission that you simply suffer from a viral infection, like the sniffles or chickenpox.

Daniel K: When I decided to go out again and actually tell my date about my problem before we had sex, the first time was the hardest. I was ner-vous as hell. And I now realize I picked someone who I thought would understand. Not just some pickup or one-nighter, so you might say I had the deck stacked in my favor. But that's another interesting thing about herpes—it changes your perspective on who you want to spend time with. I became a lot more selective.

I've also learned it's not *what* you tell someone you want to go to bed with. It's where you are mentally when you tell them. Don't get me wrong, some women have reacted negatively—politely, but negatively. But say seventy-five percent have asked me questions about it, and then went ahead and slept with me. For me, the trick is to first feel good about myself when I talk about it.

What exactly do you say?

I don't have any rules. But here are some things to keep in mind—and this should benefit anyone who is about to go out and tell someone else for the first time. Don't wait until you are both about to jump in bed. The earlier, the better; for two reasons. One, if the person reacts poorly, then you won't have to spend a lot of time being nervous and building up great expectations. And two, if the person is undecided, then he or she has the rest of the night, or weekend, or whatever, to think about it and to realize what a wonderful person you are—with or without some little virus running around in your body.

There's a great scene in Woody Allen's *Annie Hall* where he and Diane Keaton are walking down the street on their way to the movies. It's their first date, and suddenly Woody stops in the middle of the block and asks her for a kiss. It's a little awkward, and she asks him why does he want a kiss all of a sudden? He tells her that the worst part of any date—I'm paraphrasing here—is the anxiety that builds up all evening about getting a goodnight kiss. So he says he'd like to get it out of the way so he can relax and enjoy himself. I think he uses the term, "to break the ice." And, of course, she kisses him.

Is that the way it is in real life, though?

Most of the time, it's worked out well—like the woman I live with now. At first, she politely but firmly refused to go to bed with me. I was hurt, but I could see her point. I think she was a little skeptical about my ability to judge my infectiousness. She knows she's taking a calculated risk every time we make love. But we've been together for almost a year now, and we take no precautions except abstaining whenever I feel the prodrome. Most of the time, the "prodrome alert," as we call it, turns out to be a false alarm. But we don't take any chances. We might be together for a long time. I don't want to give it to her, and she doesn't want to get it. We work on it together.

Complications and How to Avoid Them

7

Keratitis and Encephalitis

My brother-in-law gets coldsores all the time and used saliva to lubricate hs contact lenses. He got a herpes infection in his eye. Thank God they caught it in time. — SHELLY M.

Herpes simplex virus does not always confine itself to the skin and mucous membranes of the nose, mouth and genitals. In its ceaseless venture to replicate, herpes simplex virus can attack the cells of the eye—and even more infrequently, the brain. But if caught in time, both of these frightening herpesvirus infections can be treated successfully. Thorough knowledge of symptoms increases the likelihood of prompt diagnosis, so it's most important to familiarize yourself with the symptoms of these two potentially destructive herpesvirus complications.

Herpes infection of the eye is called *herpes keratitis*, and may well be the most common cause of infectious blindness in the world. Though herpes keratitis is not required to be reported to federal disease and health authorities, health and pharmaceutical companies suggest that between 50,000 to 500,000 new cases occur each year. And according to another estimate, as many as 20,000 Americans lose their sight each year as a direct result of herpes keratitis. Most cases of herpes keratitis affect only one eye; only two to three percent of keratitis patients are effected bilaterally. A study done at Philadelphia's Scheie Eye Institute in conjunction with the University of Pennsylvania found that only 2 of the 1,000 patients studied ever developed ocular herpes infections.

How does someone get herpes keratitis? In two ways. One, which occurs as a biological error on the part of the migrating viral particles, happens only to people who have oral herpesvirus. On their way from the site of the original surface infection, the virions normally travel along the nerves toward the trigeminal ganglion near the temples. In very rare instances, some virions take a "wrong turn" and wind up on the nerve axon leading to the eye. The other, and far more common, way of contracting herpes keratitis is through auto-inoculation. This "self-infection" occurs when someone touches an active virus-shedding lesion (any lesion, from any person, from any part of the body) and then transfers virus particles to his or her own eye.

The eye has a mini-immune system all its own: antibacterial and anti-viral agents secreted through the tear ducts constantly bathe the eye in a protective solution. As many as half of all such infections are "curable," or at least controllable by the body's own immune system. They cause no permanent damage and do not recur. Occasionally, though, as in other immune system components, this defense fails. When this happens, infection results, most commonly in the conjunctiva, the thin membrane that lines both the inside of the eyelid and eyeball itself. Any inflammation of this mucous membrane is termed *conjunctivitis*—or to us laymen, pinkeye.

If medical help is not obtained immediately, scarring of the cornea may result. If the infection goes unchecked, it burrows deeper. If the iris is affected, it usually results in partial or total blindness—permanently. But fortunately, this form of herpesvirus is treatable (if not curable), because the eye's cellular structure permits effective application of topical drugs.

Vira-A and Stoxil are two anti-viral drugs now being used in the U.S. to combat ocular herpes infections. Extremely effective in killing the virus and stopping its spread, these topical agents are about 95 percent successful in preventing permanent damage to the eye membrane, cornea, and iris. But vision can be saved *only* if the patient is examined by an opthamologist and diagnosed in an early stage in the infection.

This is another example of how awareness and common sense can help control—if not cure—most manifestations of herpes simplex virus. Most, if not all, cases of herpetic blindness could be avoided if the patients sought treatment upon noticing the first symptoms. These are the warning signs of herpes keratis:

1. Redness of the eye.
2. Itching.
3. Irritation.
4. The feeling that there's a foreign body in the eye—which does not go away after an eyewash.
5. Discharge from the eye—either a drippy, watery liquid or a thicker mucus.
6. Swelling of the eye and surrounding tissue, resembling ordinary conjunctivitis.
7. Photophobia (unusual sensitivity to light).

Herpes eye infections occur in children as well as in adults. Those susceptible should learn the preceding symptoms and, should they suspect an infection, consult their physician immediately. Possible cases require serious attention, plus close monitoring by physicians experienced in treating keratitis. (Most forms of herpesvirus are recurrent, and herpes keratitis is no exception.) Not all symptoms need to be present, and certainly not all pinkeye infections are caused by herpesvirus. But anyone who suspects keratitis shouldn't wait to see whether it "clears up by itself." A false alarm, and subsequent reassurance by a doctor, is a far better bet.

When herpesviruses infect the brain, the disease is called *herpes simplex virus encephalitis* (HSVE). If diagnosis is not made immediately, coma, brain damage, and death ensue in most cases. This complication is exclusively restricted to people who have oral herpes infections. Again, as in herpes keratitis, the viral particle has to take a biological wrong turn: instead of going back into the trigeminal ganglion when it can become dormant, the virion follows a nerve leading back to the brain and goes on to create an infection there. One expert suggests that only 100 cases of HSVE occurred last year in the United States. In view of the 20 million or more who carry oral herpes virus, 100 cases averages out to merely 5 per million. But death occurs in about 70 percent of the patients who fail to be diagnosed accurately and treated immediately. Survivors suffer permanent damage to their brains and/or nervous systems because brain cells and nerve cells do not regenerate if injured or destroyed.

If HSVE is diagnosed in its *very early* stages, the death rate can be reduced to nearly zero, and the likelihood of permanent injury is similarly minimized. Treatment is intravenous doses of Adenine arabinoside (or Ara-A), an anti-viral drug that destroys the virus's ability to replicate and which is highly effective in early-diagnosed cases of HSVE.

Early diagnosis is essential for recovery from HSVE. Unfortunately, first symptoms are so general as to allay any real concern: headache, fever and sensitivity to light. Next to come are general malaise, muscle weakness, disorientation, and personality changes. Within a week, patients may be in a coma; days or weeks later, they may be dead. After the diagnosis of HSVE is confirmed, immediate administration of Ara-A gives excellent results. (This drug is also effective in the rare cases in which herpesvirus becomes generalized and spill into the bloodstream—an infection known as *herpetic viremia.*

Those with a history of oral herpes shouldn't panic if they feel these common cold and flu symptoms. HSVE is *extremely* rare; one has a better chance of winning the State Lottery than of falling ill with HSVE. But should you notice these symptoms in addition to feelings of uneasiness (including great disorientation, light sensitivity, and the feeling of "being a different person") then you should see a doctor.

Just as an outbreak of oral herpesvirus sometimes causes herpes encephalitis, so, in rare cases, can a genital herpesvirus infection result in a mild form of spinal meningitis. On route back to the lumbo-sacral ganglion from the site of the infection, an errant herpes virion might get into the wrong neural pathway and infect the meninges, the spine's protective membrane.

Inflammation of the meninges, either in the brain or spine, causes severe headaches, nausea, vomiting, and high fever. Neck and back muscles may spasm and prevent the patient from moving the head forward. Or the spasms may bow the patient's back backwards. Delirium may ensue and eventually coma.

If you experience any of the above symptoms, call your physician at once. In recent years, sulfa drugs and antibiotics have dramatically improved the recovery rate, which still depends upon the severity of the infection and the speed of diagnosis. Again, this information is presented not to alarm, but to make the herpesvirus patient aware of all potential complications: the chances of developing spinal meningitis in the aftermath of a genital herpesvirus is extraordinarily unlikely.

8

The Cancer Connection

An interesting aside is that every one of these cancers are reported more frequently in persons who smoke.
— WILLIAM H. WICKETT JR, MD

Cancer ranks second only to heart disease as a killer of Americans. Each year, some 25,000 American women are diagnosed as having cervical cancer—which, after breast cancer, is the most frequent malignancy in women. And biomedical research shows that women with genital herpes infections are five to eight times more likely to develop this particular condition.

Cancer, basically, is out-of-control cellular growth. From the moment of conception until death, the human organism is constantly changing: it grows, digests, excretes waste and sleeps, reacting to its environment in hundreds of different ways. In order to sustain life, cells must reproduce constantly—and perhaps as many as several million new cells are created daily. Normal cells remain organized and specialized, becoming integrated units of tissue, blood, and other organs in the body. But some cells, for reasons not yet fully understood, fail to obey the internal genetic instructions regarding growth, organization, and function. These cancer cells are abnormal in size and shape and they grow into clumps, cell upon cell in a haphazard mass.

Tumors are generally defined as swellings in or on any part of the body; growths that serve no physiological function are also known as *neoplasms*. A tumor that does not significantly invade surrounding tissue is termed benign. Sometimes, however, the bloodstream carries cells from the cancerous growth elsewhere in the body, where they find new sites to colonize. Tumors that invade surrounding tissue or contribute to secondary growths are malignant, and their unrestrained growth threatens the whole organism.

There are about 100 different kinds of cancer that affect humans, and research into its causes and cures costs more than $1 billion annually.

Researchers can describe *how* a cell behaves when it becomes cancerous, but they are unable to explain exactly why it goes awry in the first place. But after extensive scientific study, the cause-and-effect relationship between viruses and certain animal cancers is well-established. At the beginning of the 20th century, American scientist Dr. Francis P. Rous extracted a virus from the breast tumor of a Plymouth Rock hen and injected it into the breasts of ten other fowls. Within weeks, signs of cancerous growth were evident in four of the birds. Rous's work gave other scientists the impetus to pursue the viral link to cancer.

Other studies have determined the existence of viral activity in the cancers of non-human primates. In 1962, bacteriologist Dr. Bernice Eddy discovered a simian virus, SV-40, that causes cancer in monkeys—the first such virus conclusively known to cause cancer in primates. (Humans, of course, are primates too—one of the 200-odd species in this phylum.)

The viral role in *human* cancer is not so definite, however. Researchers have conducted epidemiological studies to determine whether patients infected by a particular virus are more likely to develop a specific cancer. Other investigators have analyzed the blood of cancer patients to check for the presence of antibodies, revealing which viruses the body has been exposed to, since it is often easier to detect the presence of antibodies than the viruses themselves.

Scientists seeking to prove a link between viruses and human cancer suspect that RNA and DNA viruses play a part in the process, since under electron microscope examination, many tumor cells reveal the presence of DNA and RNA viruses. Since RNA and DNA direct all cellular activity. they may also play a role in the beginnings of cancerous cellular activity. Biologist Marvin Rich has isolated an RNA virus from cells of a woman's breast tumor, and cell biologist Robert Gallo isolated another virus from the cancerous cells of a leukemia patient.

In a study conducted about twenty years ago, researchers observed that in a controlled group of thousands of women, prostitutes were found to have the highest rate of cervical cancer, and nuns the lowest incidence. This form of cancer was rare in women who had never experienced sexual intercourse with a man. From this, the researchers concluded that sexual intercourse—or at least some aspect of sexual contact—managed somehow to increase susceptibility to cervical cancer. Later studies have demonstrated that the more sex partners a woman has had, the greater her risk of cervical cancer.

Naturally enough, physicians have wondered whether cervical cancer was transmitted sexually by some infection. The first diseases they checked were syphilis and gonorrhea, but no documentable link could be uncovered. The search continued. Then evidence suggested that herpes virus can at least *contribute* to the growth of cancer in human beings. A form of neck cancer known as Burkitt's lymphoma, characterized by exceptionally fast growing cells, contains a strain of herpes known as Epstein-Barr virus (or EBV), which is also the cause of infectious mononucleosis or "mono." In the early 1960's, tumors extracted from Burkitt's lymphoma patients showed the presence of EBV. Inspired by this discovery, researchers focused on another sexually transmittable infection: herpes simplex virus.

In 1969, Drs. Rawls, Tempkins and Melnick published a paper in *The American Journal of Epidemiology* entitled, "The Association of Herpes Virus Type 2 and Carcinoma of the Uterine Cervix," detailing their study which demonstrated a high rate of cervical cancer in women who harbored HSV infections. Other research teams offered extensive and conclusive evidence that women with genital herpes infections were two to three times more likely to develop cervical cancer than women from a randomly selected control group. In addition, herpes simplex virus Type I (HSV-I) has been detected in some forms of human face, head, and neck cancer, and herpes simplex Type II (HSV-II) has been found in specimens of growths in cervical and genital areas.

Yet the discovery of any single virus lurking in a cancer cell does not necessarily prove that the virus had any role in that cancer's formation. Science has not found any hard data that cancer is contagious—as it would presumably have to be, were it caused by a contagious virus. For example, do men who have genital herpes also share a greater risk of cancer? Apparently not. Herpes simplex virus antibodies *are* found in some men who develop urogenital cancers, but only in the same proportions found in random samplings of the male population. True, the HSV-related cervical cancer studies far outnumber studies of HSV-related male urogenital cancers, and this could account for an imbalance in the statistics. But at present, the incidence of male urogenital cancer with evidence of herpes antibodies is negligible and insignificant.

Though statistical and clinical relationships between herpes and cervical cancer have been thoroughly documented, science is, again, at a loss to demonstrate that herpesvirus actually foments the growth of cancer. There's no proof, for example, that a pre-existing cervical cancer doesn't simply compromise the body's immune system, thereby making it easier for a herpes infection to take root. If cancer is in fact a "symptom" of weakened natural resistance, then it would make sense that scientists often find evidence of HSV in cervical cancer patients. And there's no reason to believe that any particular virus by *itself* can produce cancer in humans. Future research may show that cancer is a collaborative result of different factors such as radiation, environmental carcinogens, and perhaps other, currently unknown elements.

Certainly, genital herpes infection is not the only factor that increases chances of cervical cancer. Women who begin having sexual intercourse early in life, who have many different sex partners, and who have been exposed to other sexually transmittable diseases also run an above-average risk. The cause-and-effect relationship—if any—between herpes and cervical cancer has not been detected. But there is a definite *statistical* relationship: estimates suggest that about 6 percent of women who contract genital herpes will develop cervical cancer within five years. This shadowy link is responsible for much of the media attention now being focused on herpesvirus—but that's basically a good thing, because if detected early, cervical cancer is 100 percent curable.

The answer is a safe, quick, and inexpensive procedure known as a Pap smear. The name "Pap" is actually a nickname for Dr. George Papanicolaou (1883–1962) who, half a century ago, developed the technique of looking for cancer by staining and examining cells that the body has sloughed off, like the leaves on a tree, and present in secretions from the cervix and endocervical canal. A Pap smear, then, is a method of examining cells naturally shed by the lining of the cervix. Laboratory tests reveal information about these cells and in some cases, can tell a great deal about the condition of the patient in general. Pap smears are by far and away the leading method of detecting cervical cancer in its early stages—and even more important is that it can detect treatable pre-cancerous changes. Physicians estimate that the test is about 97 percent accurate.

In its initial stages, cervical cancer causes no pain at all, since the cervix has remarkably few nerve endings and the cancer begins to develop only on the most superficial lining. There are no other symptoms for the patient to perceive. But if growth continues unchecked, the malignancy will eventually invade the entire pelvic region. In such advanced stages, survival is unlikely. That's why for women with genital herpes infections, a Pap smear is *crucial*—and should be had by all women, whether afflicted with HSV or not, as part of their regular gynecological examinations.

Though a variety of methods work well, it is common practice for gynecologists to use a wooden spatula (similar to a tongue depressor) or cotton swab to lightly scrape specific regions of the cervix and vagina to collect samples of shedding cells. The Pap smear is absolutely painless—described by some patients as a feeling like the gentle scraping of a popsicle stick inside one's cheek. During pelvic exams, many women report that they don't even feel the procedure. The cells are then transferred onto a glass slide that is usually immersed in, or sprayed with, a chemical agent to preserve the cells for analysis by a laboratory technician, overseen by an M.D.

The slide is usually sent to a lab that specializes in evaluating cells and cell abnormalities. In the lab, the cells are stained to improve their visual contrast, and should a technician spot a suspicious-looking specimen, the slide is scrutinized by a staff cytopathologist—a specialist in cell pathology—before giving a report to the doctor who submitted the slide.

Once under the microscope, the slide will be assigned a grade by the technician, who watches for unusual cellular structure. A *Class I* smear is perfectly negative—no abnormal cells are observed. *Class II* shows slightly unusual cell structure, generally due to an infection—usually trichomonas, yeast, or herpes—and is not considered positive. (Some cytopathologists simply report results as "Negative" or "Positive," and include comments where appropriate.) If treatment is warranted, the physician will repeat the smear test, after the infection subsides.

Classes III, IV, and V range, respectively, from "somewhat suspicious" to "may be cancerous" to "probably cancerous." Classes IV and V are considered positive—evidence of abnormality is observed. Positive Pap smears do not prove existence of cancer in the cervix, but do alert the gynecologist to varying likelihoods of cancer.

What happens when a woman's Pap smear is graded III, IV, or V? For complete accuracy, the integrity of the Pap smear procedure must be maintained in three critical areas: the actual process of collecting the cells from the patient by the gynecologist, the application and preservation of the cells on the slide, and the microscopic evaluation of the specimen in the laboratory. If the gynecologist or cytopathologist has any doubts about the accuracy of the Pap smear results, he will repeat the procedure.

If there are no doubts about the test (or if the smear is repeated and the same results are obtained), then the doctor will perform a biopsy—a simple surgical procedure in which a small piece of tissue is removed from the cervical lining for examination under a microscope—or a coloscopy. (The coloscope is a binocular-like instrument that magnifies the surface of the cervix, enabling the physician to perform a more accurate biopsy. Membranes to be observed through the coloscope are treated with a solution that enhances the contrast of any unusual cells.) Such examinations, which are routinely performed in the doctor's office, make it possible to pinpoint the abnormal growth, improving upon the hit-or-miss quality of a random-site biopsy. These procedures are used to confirm or negate the findings of the Pap smear.

What if the biopsy or coloscopy is positive too? Courses of treatment are determined by many factors—diagnosis is only one. Whether a hysterectomy is performed depends on the patient's situation and state of mind. What are her plans for future childbearing? Sometimes treatment consists of just waiting and watching the progress of the growth. Some patients with a Class III condition are treated by having the abnormal growth cauterized. Another method of treatment is cryosurgery, which freeze-burns the growth and destroys it.

Treatment of positively proven Class IV and V conditions depends upon the stage of the disease. If biopsy indicates a malignant growth and the disease is still in an early stage of development, women who want to maintain their ability to have children need not have a complete hysterectomy—if they have early cervical cancer in which only the surface cells are involved. But if the cancer is advanced, and the malignancy has penetrated the surface layer and grown deeper into the cervical tissue, then one of the accepted treatments is a complete hysterectomy—surgical removal of the uterus and cervix. Another acceptable treatment might be local excision—removal of only the uterus or womb. Depending upon many variables, surgeons may elect to perform the operation either by a surgical incision through the abdominal wall or by proceeding through the vagina.

It's impossible to exaggerate the importance of the Pap smear, because cancer of the cervix, if detected early, is almost 100 percent curable. Fortunately, Pap smears can detect abnormal pre-cancerous cell changes up to ten years before cancer might develop. But no woman should wait that long, nor minimize the life-saving value of Dr. Papanicolaou's simple discovery. Pap smears should be taken *at least* once a year. Annually, some 10,000 American women die of cervical cancer, and the simple precaution of a Pap smear could prevent nearly every one of those fatalities. Any woman who has contracted genital herpes and reads this chapter is not likely to become one of tragic statistics—because prevention is simply too easy.

9

Herpesvirus During Pregnancy and Childbirth

When my obstetrician told me I was pregnant, he said "Keep me advised of all outbreaks and there'll be no problem."

If an infant contracts herpesvirus from its mother while being delivered, some very serious, life-threatening problems can result. Most frequently, viral particles are transmitted to an infant from active lesions in or around the mother's vagina. The virions attach themselves to cells in the eyes, nose, mouth, or in an abrasion on the skin. And the statistics are gruesome: almost seventy percent of infants who contract the virus during birth are subject to *herpetic viremia*—a massive systemic infection that becomes generalized and spreads unchecked through the entire body. More than three-quarters of these generalized infections prove fatal. Surviving infants almost invariably sustain blindness or severe damage to the brain and central nervous system. Less than five percent of those infected survive without some permanent physical damage.

Other infants, however, are spared viremia. The infection becomes localized, commonly on the eyes, mouth, nose, or areas of the skin that may have been abraded during birth—and these infants usually live. But in about half the cases of local infection, there is a high incidence of permanent damage, just as in the systemic viremic infections.

Why does herpesvirus take such a merciless toll on infants? Basically, because the human infant is born with an extremely weak immune system. When a neonate comes into the world, the only antibodies circulating in its bloodstream are those that it has acquired directly from the mother's bloodstream, via the placenta, during the fetus's nine-month stay in the womb.

Infant mortality for *all* diseases is highest during the first few weeks of life, and greatest of all during the first few days. But with each succeeding hour, the infantile immune system "learns" more about its environment. As a baby encounters antigens—as it must, by simply eating and breathing—

its system becomes sensitized to potential invaders. Though there is no precise schedule, the process of developing a complete, independent, fully-operational system of white blood cells can take from three to six months. Thereafter, the child is able to handle the virions. By the age five, most children have an immune system able to keep the virus particles "pinned down" and thus prevent viremia. In any typical kindergarten classroom (particularly during changes of season), a few children will display oral herpesvirus lesions. Unless spread to the eye, these infections are not in the least dangerous.

Even in an adult, the primary attack of herpesvirus is usually many times worse than the recurrences; the difference is that few infants survive their primary infection. But last year, physician and health authorities estimated that no more than 1,000 live births resulted in viremic herpesvirus. Compared to the 3.4 million live births annually in the United States, this statistic does not seem terribly frightening; the problems seems fairly well under control. But the epidemic proportions of genital herpesvirus infections among adults increases the risk of neonatal herpesvirus. What worries public health officials is the extrememly high incidence of genital herpesvirus in women of childbearing age—and the fact that the infected population continues to increase. Through awareness, however, it's likely that the number of infected infants can be reduced dramatically—to perhaps only a handful of cases annually. Just as with cervical cancer, cooperation with an alert physician can all but eliminate some of herpesvirus's most serious aspects.

Even if a woman has vaginal herpes infections during her pregnancy, it's not likely for the fetus to contract the virus through the placenta unless she develops viremia—and normal adults rarely become viremic during a herpesvirus recurrence. But a pregnant woman with a *primary* outbreak of herpesvirus does run a greater risk of the virus spilling into her bloodstream and infecting the amniotic fluid. There is a case on record in which the amniotic fluid showed signs of herpesvirus infection, yet the infant when delivered was perfectly healthy. Although reason for this good fortune is not known, it further reduces the need to worry about trans-placental infections. Nevertheless, any pregnant woman with a history of genital herpesvirus infection should inform her obstetrician. When you work together with a concerned, alert physician, the chances for any herpesvirus complications are extremely small. And if your doctor does not take an active, *aggressive* interest in your history of herpesvirus, you should get another doctor.

First, the physician will want to make sure that the infection you complain about is really herpesvirus.

Methods of Diagnosis

About 95 percent of genital herpesvirus infections are diagnosed by a physician's clinical observation of the lesions. The characteristic appearance of a herpesvirus sore, together with the patient's symptoms and history, paint a rather clear picture of the infection for the doctor. But there may be mitigating circumstances. When a pregnant woman is threatening premature delivery, and when there's the possibility of several concurrent infections, doctors like to determine exactly what might crop up. And so the examining physician may prefer to verify the clinical observation through laboratory analysis.

It is important that any laboratory test meet three criteria: it must be accurate and sensitive to the specific condition being tested for; be easily accessible to the clinicians who require the test; and yield results in a reasonably short period of time. In terms of accuracy, positive identification of herpes is best accomplished by the painless procedure of taking a culture—simply planting a sample of microorganisms and seeing what grows. To take a culture, a doctor or lab technician removes a bit of fluid from an active lesion—before the scab-like crusting occurs—and inserts it into a salt solution. The particles are then transported to the lab in that solution, where they are transferred into a culture of living cells, maintained as close as possible to 98.6° F. Like cells from the patient's body, these living cells make appropriate hosts for the suspected viral invaders. Sometimes these culture cells are from human lung tissue or from embryonic organs; cells from other species, such as chickens, are also used. (These cells, by the way, are seldom freshly extracted, but are usually the living descendents of cells obtained from "donor" organisms and cultured for laboratory purposes.)

Should the specimen contain any virus particles, they will replicate—and since viruses can replicate with great speed, the process of "seeing what grows" takes only about forty-eight hours. When herpes replication is observed, the preliminary diagnosis of herpesvirus is confirmed and the culture is labelled positive. If no viruses can be detected, then the culture is considered negative—at least from the lesion from which the specimen was taken.

But as with most tests, the possibility of incorrect results always exists —either through human error, from contaminated materials, or from a combination of the two. Physicians who make decisions for a course of clinical action always bear in mind the possibility of a falsely negative reading. And specifically, the trouble with confirming herpesvirus by culturing is the difficulty of obtaining the specimen.

Culturing is usually informative only during an outbreak; and so your doctor should arrange for the test to be performed whenever you experience your next recurrence. If you rarely or never have recurrences, there are other procedures to help the doctor ascertain whether you are subject to herpesvirus infections. Time is crucial! Unless a specimen is extracted during the active stage of viral shedding, the lab results may be falsely negative. And sometimes a negative reading is given, not because the virus wasn't present in the specimen, but because the storage and transportation of the particles in the saline solution destroyed their viability.

If a culture shows that herpesvirus *is* present, your doctor must determine whether herpesvirus particles will be present during delivery. An important factor is an accurate estimation of the baby's due date. This is crucial, because as you approach term, the culturing process must be repeated—sometimes frequently—to be sure that there is no "silent shedding" of virus particles from the skin or mucous membrane surfaces. You must keep your physician abreast of any recurrences, of lesions in sites where you have had no lesions before, and of your patterns of infection (and your husband's, if he is also infected).

Some couples find that sexual intercourse can induce recurrences—whether by friction created in the genital tract, the excitement, or the anxiety associated with sex. If a woman knows she is prone to recurrences resulting from the act of making love, then it would be wise for her to postpone intercourse well before the anticipated time of delivery.

Culturing takes about 48 hours, however, and in the case of a woman about to give birth who thinks she feels the familiar herpesvirus prodrome in her vagina, often a few hours can be too long to wait. A less accurate, but much speedier test for herpesvirus is obtained from the common Pap smear—a technique that is sometimes used when a patient suspects a genital herpesvirus infection, but displays no symptoms. But unless the Pap smear is treated specifically to "read" for herpesvirus, the virus cannot be observed.

When the life of an infant about to be born depends on the speedy evaluation of a possible herpes lesion, electron microscopy is unquestionably the fastest way to detect the presence of herpesvirus, although only specialized labs have electron microscopes, owing to their fantastic cost. (A modest model can easily cost $85,000 and the fancier electron microscopes are priced in the hundreds of thousands.) Another problem is that as seen through the electron microscope, all members of the herpes family have the same shape. The herpes zoster virus, which causes shingles and chickenpox, looks similar to the Epstein-Barr virus; and one cannot positively distinguish a herpes simplex virus. But since no other herpesvirus causes symptoms that parallel those of herpes simplex, it's logically assumed that any herpesvirus viral particle obtained from a genital lesion *has* to be a herpes simplex virus. Despite these drawbacks, electron microscopy offers an excellent advantage. Once a fraction of a drop of vesicular fluid is subjected to EM examination, the results are practically immediate: diagnosis can be made within fifteen to twenty minutes.

If the tests show herpesvirus is present and if your doctor believes that herpesvirus particles will be present at the expected time of delivery, he or she will likely recommend a Caesarean section (surgical delivery through the abdomen).

But even though positive cultures may have been obtained only weeks before the due date of vaginal delivery, a C-section is not necessarily assured. When cultures of areas prone to lesions (or crusty areas of a recent lesion) show no presence of the virus, vaginal deliveries are generally permitted. Since Caesarean sections carry some risk of complications and morbidity to both fetus and mother, unnecessary Caesareans should be avoided whenever possible. Of course, the women who have been subject to continuous, or almost continuous genital herpesvirus infections should not risk vaginal delivery, but the final determination of method of birth will usually not be made until the onset of labor.

Whenever Caesarean section is deemed appropriate, the procedure should be performed electively—that is, at the doctor's discretion, rather than after labor has begun and spontaneous birth appears imminent. Studies show that if such a procedure is carried out before the fetal membrane is ruptured, chances of infection are minute. Chances of infection are still low if the time elapsed since the membrane ruptured remains less than four hours.

As soon as the doctors determine that the neonate has no herpesvirus infection, all procedures are normal. However, if there is even the slightest suspicion that there may have been infection, the infant will be isolated from other newborns and monitored closely (though there are no truly effective treatments at this time).

Babies can also contract herpesvirus *postpartum* from a parent, hospital staff member, friend or sibling who is shedding virus particles at the time. Since an infant seldom contracts herpesvirus through its own healthy, unbroken skin—an excellent barrier that easily excludes most viral and bacterial invaders—the most common sites of infection are the mucous membranes. Kissing is particularly dangerous because it may transfer a virus particle directly to mucous membranes on the infant's mouth, nose, or eye. Also, an infant is prone to reach out and touch adults' faces (where virus particles may be present), and then return the hand to its mouth. Parents should take careful hygienic precautions, including frequent hand washing whenever lesions are apparent anywhere on the parent's body. Adults and children with active lesions should be kept away from the infant entirely.

Fighting
Back

10

"Cures" That Don't Work

*It is better to know nothing than to know
what ain't so.* — JOSH BILLINGS, *Affurisms*

The U.S. Department of Health and Human Services, through its Centers for Disease Control, has published a pamphlet entitled *Ineffective Therapies for Genital Herpes Infections*, subtitled "Don't Harm Yourself with Treatments That Don't Work." In an introduction to the pamphlet, the Department issues this warning:

> At present, no drug, vaccine, diet or treatment has shown to be effective in preventing recurrences of genital *Herpes simplex* infections. Several locally-applied preparations may relieve the discomfort of herpes, but none changes the course of the disease.

The pamphlet goes on to describe twenty-six different treatments, none of which has been proven effective. Many of these treatments are topical medications applied to the surface of the skin:

- *Betadine* is an iodine-based microbial antiseptic good for cleansing wounds and preventing secondary infections, but it is not at all worthwhile in destroying herpesvirus or in healing lesions that are already established.
- *DMSO*, or dimethyl sulfoxide, a skin-penetrating solvent, has been credited with curing everything from acne to cancer. Available over the counter in many states, it is often mixed with anti-viral compounds and applied to herpesvirus lesions. But in terms of safety, DMSO is an unproven substance. (The reason it's so readily available is because the FDA does not classify it as a drug or medicine!) Experimentation with it is definitely not recommended.
- *Dye-light therapy:* In the early 1970s, a group of Houston researchers sent a wave of excitement through the medical world by reporting that they had found an effective method of treating herpesvirus infections in the eyes of rabbits. Their remedy was relatively simple: lesions caused by herpesvirus were swabbed with a light-sensitive dye, believed to

be absorbed by viral DNA. When exposed to ultraviolet light waves, this special dye made the virus stop replicating.

The technique caught on and was soon being used all across the country to treat herpesvirus outbreaks. Then in 1973, Dr. Fred Rapp of the Pennsylvania State University College of Medicine reported that this treatment was not only ineffective, but dangerous as well: the dye could potentially cause cancer in uninfected cells. In 1975, a research group at the Harvard Medical School divulged the results of their own study of the dye-light treatment: it did not hasten the healing of herpesvirus lesions, nor did it reduce the frequency or severity of recurring infections. Furthermore, some cases of Bowen's disease, a cancer of the penis, have now been attributed to dye-light therapy. So if you had to pick one treatment to avoid, this would seem to be it.

- *Ether* was once thought to cripple the virus's ability to replicate. Applying ether to the sores was recommended by Albert Sabin, M.D., the man who developed the polio vaccine, and his stature in the medical world lent credence to his claim. Unfortunately, subsequent studies found that ether was ineffective. Although ether is an anesthetic, it causes a painful burning sensation when applied to herpesvirus lesions—one more reason why this treatment is no longer in favor.

- *Laser surgery* has also been touted as an "instant total release from herpes recurrences. Over a 14-month period, Dr. Michael Truppin of New York's Mount Sinai Hospital cauterized the herpesvirus sores of some 115 women who were experiencing genital infections. When lesions continued to appear after two weeks of treatment, the laser therapy was discontinued—but was considered a success when patients did not have further recurrences within a 12-month period. According to *The Helper*, "Dr. Truppin . . . stated that better results were obtained when the treatment was administered within 48 hours after lesions appeared in the primary [infection] and that recurrences were less responsive to this technique." This makes sense, since the virions in a *primary* lesion might not have had time to invade the nerve pathways.

"Truppin cautions that . . . in his own practice, this treatment is limited to those with severe disease symptoms," And *The Helper* adds "it must be emphasized that laser therapy has no effect on the latent virus."

- *Lithium:* the popular press has reported that a substance known as lithium carbonate has been effective in diminishing recurrences of genital herpesvirus infections. These reports, regrettably, are not confirmed. Although research *may* eventually show lithium to be an important antiherpesvirus agent, its powers (if any) have yet to be substantiated. Further controlled tests are in order before lithium can be prescribed as an effective anti-herpes drug.

There are isolated reports of people who have tried treating themselves with illicit lithium carbonate—which seems not to be a very smart idea. Lithium is an intensely powerful compound with a wide range of damaging side effects including (but not limited to) disorientation, convulsions, and kidney disease. Some deaths have even been attributed to inadequately supervised lithium carbonate treatment.

- *Silcadene* is usually applied to halt bacterial infections in patients ⸱ been badly burned, but it has no demonstrable effect upon and certainly doesn't kill the virus particles.

nacides kill spermatozoa, but have no ill effects on herpes- they often irritate sensitive skin (particulary new tissue , healing) and retard the formation of new, healthy cells.

id creams such as mycalog are sometimes prescribed to prevent ᴏ.........ate secondary infections at the site of herpesvirus lesions. These creams do help reduce the itching and burning sensations of inflamed tissue, but frequently irritate the skin and actually inhibit the healing of lesions.

Vaccines

Science knows of no vaccine that is able to protect those who are as yet uninfected with herpesvirus. and because vaccines are used to *prevent* diseases, not treat them, the vaccine for any other virus is not about to stimulate the immune system to produce anitbodies against herpesvirus— though it may possibly boost the immune system as a whole. Actually, the use of *any* vaccine bears certain risks; vaccines have been so widely used only because the alternatives—diseases such as polio, tuberculosis, smallpox, and others—are so much worse. Since no vaccine has any demonstrable effect in helping boost antibodies against herpesvirus, it is dangerous to use them for that purpose.

In 1979, in a study at the University of Alabama Medical Center, great quantities of *Influenza virus vaccine* (IVV) were injected into patients with herpesviurs infections. Since the injected viruses are not alive, IVV is particularly safe and free of side effects. Results were dramatic, but again, the study was not thoroughly controlled—and IVV is not being used until further controlled studies can be evaluated.

- *Lupidon G*, a German vaccine, has been used in Europe, but has not yet been approved for use in the U.S. Although it is touted as being specifically effective in recurring cases of genital herpesvirus infections, there is no evidence that Lupidon G works as claimed.

- *Yellow-fever vaccine* has been used infrequently in the treatment of herpesvirus, but has absolutely no effect on infections caused by the virus. This vaccine's only known application is against yellow fever.

Not all vaccines are created—some are quite literally born. Two French scientists, Calmette and Guerin, had cultured generation after generation of tuberculosis bacteria. Somehow, a few of the bacilli mutated into organisms that, under a microscope, look and behave like ordinary tuberculosis, but do not cause disease symptoms! When injected into human beings, this strain, now called Bacillus Calmette–Guerin (or BCG), successfully immunized them against tuberculosis.

For many years, researchers had reason to hope that BCG acted as a non-specific immune stimulator—that is, that it stimulated the immune system into becoming more aggressive in general, not just toward the tuberculosis bacilli specifically. Many herpesvirus patients are aware of a University of California at Los Angeles experiment using BCG to reduce the frequency and severity of recurrences. Results were marginally favorable, but the study was criticized for being uncontrolled. Subsequent controlled tests of BCG on herpesvirus patients showed, however, that the BCG had no effect. Further research indicated that BCG does improve immune response—in some individuals. But there also seem to be some negative side effects. One study seeking to evalutate BCG's ability to affect immune response observed that in some laboratory animals injected with BCG, cancer tumors grew faster than in control animals—all of which has disconcerting implications for the possible effects of BCG on the human immune system.

The Placebo Effect

In terms of scientifically reproducible studies, the Health Department pamphlet is technically correct that the therapies it describes "are of no proven value in the treatment of genital herpes." While patients should not treat themselves with any untested, potentially toxic substance, there are many herpesvirus sufferers who would debate the Health Department's claim that "none changes the course of the disease." Some patients swear by one or more of the treatments that the pamphlet says don't work. The success they experience may be due to those individuals' specific metabolic make-up—or because of the well-known placebo effect. A good example is the experience of Tim A., who caught genital herpesvirus at the Mardi Gras in New Orleans when he was 21 years old.

> Tim: *As soon as I got back to school, I noticed an itching and redness on my penis. I didn't know what the hell it was. I was plenty worried so I immediately went to the college infirmary. The doctor knew what it was right away and gave me some green junk to put on it. I didn't know about herpes then, and didn't ask any questions. I just put the stuff on, and the infection went away. In the following months, it came back a few times and I just used the cream like I did the first time. Well, I was*

almost out of the stuff, and school was about to break, so I asked the doctor for another tube for the summer. He told me that he had a new medicine that would knock out the infection once and for all. This stuff was white. He said to put it on now, for the next three days, and then I wouldn't be troubled by it anymore.

I took his advice, and, believe it or not, I didn't have a recurrence for two years—until I read that nothing *could rid you of herpes; there was no way to get rid of it. Then—about three or four days after reading that, I got a tiny infection, much smaller than the others. But no way I was angry with that doctor. Actually, he was smarter than me and helped me to have a herpes-free two years. It* did *work. Now I just have to find some way to trick myself again.*

The word *placebo* in Latin means "I shall please." Science uses placebos in double-blind testing of new drugs. For example, in a double-blind, placebo-controlled study, one group of subjects takes the drug or form of treatment under investigation by the research team. Another group—known as the control group—takes a placebo, or "dummy" medication that has no biological effect at all. Frequently the placebo drug is simply a sugar pill or a saline solution, whose only purpose is to convince the participant that he's taking a "real" medicine. The subjects of these two groups do not know whether they are getting the real drug or the placebo—and for that matter, nor do the researchers themselves know who's receiving what until after the trials are completed. But well-documented medical case histories have shown that people have actually been healed from *real* illness following the prescription of a placebo. In his research paper called "Factors Contributing to the Placebo Effect" (*American Journal of Psychotherapy*, 1961), Dr. Arthur K. Shapiro, who has long studied the mind-body relationship, wrote: "placebos can have profound effects on organic illness—including incurable malignancies."

In 1960, *New Yorker* Magazine medical writer Berton Rouche wrote that placebos are effective only because of "the infinite capacity of the human mind for self-deception." But author Norman Cousins believes a mind-body alliance accomplishes the real healing. In his wonderful book *Anatomy of an Illness*, Cousins reflects upon the human mind's role in healing and regeneration:

> The doctor knows that it is the prescription slip itself, even more than what is written on it, that is often the vital ingredient for enabling a patient to get rid of whatever is ailing him. Drugs are not always necessary, belief in recovery always is.

Without a personal, sympathetic patient-doctor relationship, placebos fail to have the dramatic effects so often discovered. Thus, apparently, it is the doctor who really mobilizes the patients' ability to heal themselves. In achieving a positive result in healing, confidence, trust, and faith are crucial factors. Science has shown the debilitating physical reactions to emotions like fear, anxiety, and paranoia, but so far has been unable to document the wide range of health-inducing biochemical changes that also result from simple thought.

In a 1981 *Science Digest* article entitled "Power of the Empty Pill," writer Laurence Cherry quotes Dr. David Sobel, medical director on the Institute for the Study of Human Knowledge in San Jose, California, as saying, "The placebo response is one of the most remarkable of all medical phenomena. Now we have to learn how to harness it properly and use it to our best advantage."

Anti-Viral Drugs

Normally, doctors treat virus infections symptomatically, giving you something for the aches and fever, while letting your body do the job of putting down the invader. *Anti-viral drugs* are substances that interfere with viral particles' growth and reproduction. The trouble is that most anti-viral drugs fail to discriminate between infected cells and healthy ones—so that all the cells in their path tend to be damaged or even killed.

• *Idoxuridine (IDU)* was first used to effectively arrest herpesvirus eye infections, thereby preventing scarring of the retina and subsequent blindness. This drug comes in both solution and ointment forms and works only because eye tissue is structurally different from the labial and genital mucous membranes where herpes usually makes its home. On infections outside the eye, this product has no effect at all.

• *Inosiplex* trips up the virus in its attempts to affix its RNA to the genetic material of a host cell. An early study of Inosiplex's effects on oral and genital herpesvirus was encouraging. But as is the case with all antiviral drugs, extensive further studies must be conducted.

• *Ribavirin*, an oral anti-viral drug approved for study in the U.S., is yet another substance that inhibits viruses from successfully reprogramming the genes of a captured cell. Laboratory tests show that Ribavirin has some effectiveness in reducing replication in many viruses, including herpesvirus. But as with many such drug experiments, tests conducted in the lab or *in vitro* (in glass, as in a test tube) do not always display the same results as experiments on patients. Current experiments have been aimed at learning more about its effects on shingles, which is caused by herpes zoster. No effect was observed in persons with genital herpesvirus infections. This drug has been used experimentally on humans in trials outside the United States, in which it demonstrated some usefulness as a topical agent, but the results of ongoing tests will have to be examined before it can be licensed for use in this country.

• *Vidarabine* (better known by its popular name of *Ara-A*) is an effective treatment for eye infection—but it doesn't *cure* herpesvirus. The patient with keratitis is subject to recurrent infections, in which case further treatment with the drug is the prescribed therapy. Ara-A also has a dramatic effect on encephalitis, which less than a decade ago was an often fatal infection.

Some patients obtain prescriptions for excessive amounts of these drugs, mistakingly believing that if they halt infections on the eyes and brain, they will surely work on infections elsewhere. But Vidarabine has not been shown to have any beneficial effects in cases of oral or genital herpesvirus infections. The molecular nature of Ara-A makes it difficult to introduce into the human body, and once in the system, the drug is transformed into a less potent viral adversary. Like IDU, Ara-A has proven to be ineffective in oral and genital herpesvirus infections. But the major problem with Ara-A lies in its dangerous side effects—it damages the genes of healthy, uninfected cells and thus increases the possibility of birth defects.

At the center of all viral replication is the "blueprint" that the virus forces upon the invaded cell. Substances like Ara-A and IDU chemically "confuse" the virus's DNA and RNA, causing it to substitute a blueprint that won't build more virus particles. But many laboratory studies have demonstrated that merely disturbing viral DNA and RNA molecules is not enough to stop herpesvirus from infecting new cells. Moreover, these viral-replication inhibitors are not completely specific to the herpesvirus, and so they sometimes confuse the genetic material of normal cells—a risky situation, because a mutant cell with no real function in the body may become cancerous, continuing to divide and reproduce.

The ultimate goal of present studies and tests is to find a substance that will act specifically against cells invaded by viruses, without affecting uninfected cells in any significant way. Thus, anti-viral research is progressing in two directions: some drugs are being sought to stimulate the natural immune system against viruses in general, while others are being designed to inhibit viral replication. A major effort is under way to develop viral-replication inhibitors that possess specificity, or the ability to attack only infected cells.

11

New Treatments and Therapies

---

*There are a thousand hacking at the branches of evil
to one who is striking at the root.*
— HENRY DAVID THOREAU, *Walden*

Scientists at the University of Michigan, headed by Dr. Charles Shipman, announced in the summer of 1982 that they had met with dramatic success in their studies of a complex chemical known as *acetylpyridine thiosemicarbazone.* Shipman stated in a *Time* Magazine article that the substance "has a potency hundreds of times greater than that of drugs currently used" in the treatment of primary and recurrent herpes simplex virus infections. Though the drug does not prevent recurrences, the scientists claim it is effective against development of the herpesvirus lesion once the infection begins.

A new generation of Ara-A improvements is being developed to reduce the side effects and make dosages easier to administer. Perhaps the most promising of these new substances is called *Vidarabine monophosphate*, which is expected to be applied in cases of neonatal herpesvirus infection.

One of several optimistic developments in the effort to conquer viruses in general, and herpesvirus in particular, is *Acyclovir* or *ACV;* which was the very first drug to be approved by the FDA as a topical treatment in genital herpesvirus infections. Originally known as BW 248–U, it was developed by a group of researchers at the North Carolina laboratories of the pharmaceutical giant Burroughs Wellcome. In 1978, the FDA approved clinical tests of four different formulas of it.

The popular press has tried to explain the way acyclovir works by suggesting that it makes the herpesvirus commit suicide—an oversimplification, and a poor analogy. In fact, acyclovir sabotages the viral genes, loading the herpesvirus particles with blanks instead of live ammunition. Acyclovir's molecular structure is quite similar to thymidine kinase, a certain enzyme that the virus needs to replicate, and the herpesvirus often fails to distinguish between the two. In a sense, the herpesvirus is tricked into using the drug instead of the proper enzyme. Then, after incorporating the counterfeit enzyme into its genetic structure, the virus tries to replicate, but finds that it is genetically incomplete.

The beauty of acyclovir is that the enzyme it imitates is found *only* in cells that have been invaded by viruses. Normal, uninfected cells will not contain that enzyme, nor will they seek to acquire the ACV. (As we have seen, other anti-viral agents often fail to have such a specific effect and often damage healthy cells or, even worse, cause them to mutate.) Another important feature of this compound is its apparent lack of toxicity. High doses have been injected into laboratory animals without any negative side effects. ACV is also unaffected by the process of digestion, so that convenient oral dosages are expected to be just as effective as hypodermic injections.

Acylovir has an effect on other viruses besides herpes simplex and herpes zoster; it is also reported to be effective against mononucleosis. Burroughs Wellcome estimates that acyclovir is about one hundred times more effective than Ara-A, the major competing anti-viral compound. Though its efficacy in reducing the severity of genital infections remains to be seen, the drug has an undisputed effect on viral replication in immunocompromised patients harboring herpesvirus. In a well-controlled clinical test of 20 bone-marrow transplant candidates, 10 patients received a placebo and 10 received ACV intravenously. Later, when the researchers "broke the code" imposed upon the experiment to assure strict objectivity, they found that 75 percent of the patients receiving the placebo had developed oral or genital herpesvirus infections, while *none* of the patients receiving ACV showed any positive culture for herpesvirus. Interestingly, when administration of ACV was stopped, several of these patients then developed infections.

Maurice Hilleman, developer of the vaccines for mumps and Hepatitis B, has stated, "Acyclovir is an amazing development in that it is so specific against herpesvirus. I am truly excited." And Hilleman is employed by Merck, Sharpe, and Dohme—a competitor of the firm that manufactures ACV! As of this writing, Burroughs Wellcome is actually marketing its acyclovir product within the United States under the brand name of Zovirax for use in genital and oral herpesvirus infections. Currently available in 15-gram tubes, Zovirax is recommended to be applied topically up to four times a day. Physicians are administering it in the following ways:

1. As a petroleum-base ointment for herpes keratitis.
2. As a topical ointment for oral and genital infections.
3. As an orally-ingested drug for both herpes simplex virus and herpes zoster (shingles).

4. As an intravenous solution for extremely serious herpesvirus infections and for those patients whose immune systems are naturally deficient or immunosuppressed.

According to *The Wall Street Journal*, Zovirax ointment was approved for commercial use in March of 1982. Though the FDA recommended it only for patients with first-time infections, the medicine quickly won a reputation as an effective treatment for genital herpesvirus. Later, however, a study published in the *New England Journal of Medicine* found that use of the treatment at the beginning of an initial episode reduced healing time to 10.9 days from 14.3 days, and shortened the contagious period from 7 to 4.1 days. For patients with recurring herpesvirus, the drug reduced the contagious period in men from 2.3 to 1.2 days, and in women, from 1.4 down to 0.6 days. Healing time in men was "reduced slightly," the *Medical Letter* reported, noting that it had no such effect in women. Thus while Zovirax does speed healing and reduce contagion, it is by no means a preventive measure—much less a cure.

The Promise of Interferon

Physicians have long observed the interesting fact that patients who have come down with a viral infection very rarely contract *another* viral illness at the same time. Apparently, the presence of one virus in the system somehow prevents other viruses from taking hold.

In 1965, two London scientists, Jean Lindenmann and Alick Isaacs, probed that phenomenon by infecting the membrane of a fertilized egg first with influenza virus, then with other viruses. Once the influenza had begun to replicate, no other viruses could make much headway.

Did the first virus to arrive somehow "stake its claim," making it difficult for other viral particles to invade the host? The scientists extracted infected cells containing influenza virus from the eggshell membrane. They then added healthy cells to this extract, and tried to infect them with another virus—but failed. They concluded that the original infected cells of the eggshell membrane had produced a substance that had somehow interfered with a virus's ability to attack new cells. From this characteristic of the unusual substance came its name—*interferon*.

We now know that when a virus invades a cell, it triggers the biochemical equivalent of a burglar alarm, dispatching a chemical message to protect cells from viral infection by alerting them to the presence of a specific antigen. The "messenger" is a protein known as interferon. Biochemists have isolated three different kinds of interferon that all do basically the same thing. As soon as an infected cell secretes the substance, it passes out through the cell membrane and chemically signals surrounding cells to produce anti-viral substances appropriate for whatever specific antigen the interferon has "described."

Interferon fits the profile of the ideal anti-viral (and anti-herpesvirus) agent: it is of low toxicity, reduces the chances of genetic mutation and dangerous side effects, successfully inhibits replication in all viruses, and is specific enough to spare normal cells. Perhaps nature's most potent natural inhibitor of viral attacks on cells, it may well be to viruses what penicillin is to bacteria. *Time* Magazine's cover story on interferon in March of 1980 concluded that should interferon only partly fulfill its early promise, it would still be a significant advancement. But some scientists feel that the high hopes for this substance are too good to be true and have nicknamed it IF. *Time* reported that skeptical researchers doubt that the data about interferon's capabilities are being analyzed objectively and have referred to the interferon excitement as "misinterpreton."

The major obstacle in testing interferon is the unbelievable expense involved in obtaining it from the cells that naturally produce it—in infinitesimally small quantities. Some educated guesses suggest that a pound of molecularly pure interferon could cost from between fifteen and twenty billion dollars! Many major pharmaceutical companies are investing tremendous capital to find economically feasible ways to produce the quantities of interferon that the market will require should it be proven an effective antiviral substance, much less a cancer cure.

One promising way is through recombinant DNA. The common bacillus *E. coli*, which normally inhabits the human digestive tract, can be refitted with new genes to radically alter its behavior. Recently, recombinant engineers have succeeded in creating an artificial mutation of *E. coli* that produces interferon as a byproduct of its life processes. If these little bacilli can be induced to multiply and continue to do their thing (in the gut of a patient or, better yet, *in vitro*), then interferon may become plentiful enough to facilitate widespread experimentation. Still other processes under development may reduce the cost of interferon to about 5 percent of its current level.

Other researchers are experimenting with methods to produce IF within the body *without* the help of *E. coli*—just as nature intended. Biochemists at the National Institute of Health have developed a substance known as an interferon-inducer. This chemical, called IC:LC, possesses some of the characteristics of the antigens that would normally stimulate cells to produce interferon—and it does seem to have that very effect upon cells. But as with many drugs, its use results in some negative side effects—so while it is being refined and adapted, the FDA authorities who approve new drugs must carefully weigh the substantiated benefits against the possible dangers. IC:LC has not yet been tried on humans (the final step before a drug can be licensed for general distribution), but it has climbed well towards the top of the ladder of safety and experimentation and is being tested on primates.

Similar to IC:LC are the *immunopotentiators*, substances that stimulate the body's natural immune system and have wide application for many diseases, not simply virus infections. The initial interest in immunopotentiators arose during the search for a treatment for the immuno-deficient—people whose immune systems are not working properly. Doctors believed that one or more of the immune system components was defective, and immunopotentiators were developed to bring the subnormal immune systems back in line.

Isoprinosine is an interesting anti-viral immunopotentiator that helps cells stimulate interferon production, retards viral replication, and contributes to cellular immunity. But it has thus far failed to prove its effectiveness against herpesvirus infections. This substance has a wide range of side effects, and is currently being used only experimentally.

A more widely known substance in this category is *Levamisole*, an orally ingested chemical that may be able to stimulate the immune system against all types of disease. Levamisole has been proven to enhance the immune systems of laboratory animals and bring them up to normal if their systems were chronically depressed. In early tests on children, the drug *seemed* to have a general beneficial effect, quickening recovery from a wide variety of viral diseases, including measles, influenza and respiratory infections. Though Levamisole looked like a potential success in anti-viral drug research, numerous studies since have uncovered no effect in enhancing the body's specific ability to cope with virus infections—and a number of unpleasant side effects have come to light that greatly reduce the chances of its future success. The drug commonly lowers the white blood count, leaving many patients nauseous, dizzy, and disoriented. In a controlled study of the effects of Levamisole on recurrent genital herpesvirus infections, the results indicated no beneficial effects.

Phosphonacetic Acid, or *PAA* is of special interest because it demonstrates specificity toward herpesviruses—a fundamental ingredient in any effective treatment. With specificity, it is possible to destroy the viral particles without damaging healthy, uninfected cells. Thus, PAA doesn't raise the risk of birth defects, as do IDU and Ara-A. Another feature of this interesting compound is that its toxicity is extremely low—which has induced researchers to probe further into its potential as an anti-herpesvirus agent.

Sadly, the politics of the pharmaceutical industry are such that very simple compounds such as PAA may not be patented, and so offer a manufacturing company no protection from competition, and no guarantee of profit. Some of the tests and experiments needed to win FDA approval are extremely expensive, and a single company may be reluctant to spend millions of dollars to prove that a common, naturally-occuring substance is safe and effective. Upon that drug's approval by the FDA, any other drug manufacturer could begin to package and market it, without having participated in the costly pre-approval testing program. Additionally, PAA's application is limited to the herpes simplex virus. Despite this, Abbott Labs of Chicago has initiated a PAA research program and expects to report its initial results in the early to mid-1980s.

2–deoxy–D–glucose: A cooperative research project on this compound conducted by the University of Pennsylvania and Philadelphia's Scheie Eye Institute resulted in dramatic statistics. 2–DG, as it's popularly known, is a naturally-occuring sugar easily synthesized from glucose.

More than twenty years ago, experiments measuring the effects of 2–DG on mice harboring viral influenza did not prove promising, and so this substance was not examined again for more than ten years. Then, Dr. Herbert Blough, one of the researchers now at the forefront of 2–DG investigation, reported in the medical periodicals that 2–DG had accomplished the all-important task of disturbing a virus particle's ability to make its host cell fuse with another uninfected cell. In creating this fusion, virus particles avoid the immune system components such as macrophages and the anti-viral chemicals produced by T-lymphocytes.

While other anti-viral agents inhibit replication by interfering with the herpesvirus's mechanism of transferring its genetic instructions into the host cell, 2–DG acts upon viruses by compromising the viral and cellular synthesis of sugar molecules. Lacking the full range of sugar molecules, either on its own surface or on the cell walls, the virus is unable to attach itself to the potential host cell and is, therefore, barred from transferring its genetic material. Accordingly, no viral replication can occur. The rate of infection diminishes and ultimately stops. In addition, 2–DG causes herpes-virus particles to develop without the caspid, the envelope of protein molecules they need to survive.

Theoretically, then, 2–DG should be an effective inhibitor of viral replication. In the June 29, 1979 *Journal of the American Medical Association,* Drs. Herbert Blough and Robert Giuntoli reported that in their program, 89 percent of the women treated with 2–DG upon their first outbreak of herpesvirus never had a recurring infection. 65 percent of the control group were also spared recurrences. But according to Drs. Blough and Giuntoli, in cases of recurrent herpesvirus infections, the healing rate was twice as fast as normally. Of those patients with a history of recurrent infections, 60 percent of those treated with 2–DG never had another recurrence during the 24-month post-treatment monitoring period. But the University of Pennsylvania/Scheie Eye Institute study has been roundly criticized for its apparent lack of control and its small number of subjects.

Since their 1979 report, Drs. Giuntoli and Blough have continued their treatment program, broadening it to include men and amassing data on some 1,000 people with primary and recurrent herpesvirus infections. Recently Dr. Giuntoli stated that though the results do not come from controlled, double-blind studies, they remain remarkably true to the original findings culled from the original "subject universe" of only 51 women. Should these same statistics be reproduced by other researchers in turn, it would make 2–deoxy–D–glucose one of the most exciting anti-herpesvirus substances yet known to science

This would-be wonder drug has its vociferous detractors, however. Some respected researchers claim that 2–DG cannot do what it is supposed to. And one woman believes that after she participated in the 2–DG trials, her moderate case of genital herpes became violent and severe. But certainly, future controlled tests should reveal conclusively whether 2–DG is the wonder substance that herpesvirus patients are waiting for.

One of the more popular myths about herpesvirus goes something like this: *Medical science is on the verge of a cure, and one will be discovered within the next few months.* Such is the popular faith in modern medicine that many herpesvirus patients simply can't believe that a cure doesn't already exist. But at the moment, such wishful thinking is simply unrealistic. Some researchers refer to herpesvirus as "the ultimate parasite" because of its ability to escape the immune system by hiding within the nerve pathways and ganglia. For this single reason, herpesvirus presents a genuine challenge to medicine.

We asked Sam Knox of the Herpes Resource Center if people should expect to see a cure for herpesvirus in the immediate future.

> Knox: *Based on the research that's going on today, I doubt that a complete cure will be forthcoming in the next few years. Oh, we hear of new research all the time. And many are tantalizing in their claims. But it's a basic precept of biomedical research that results must be reproducible by other researchers. We hope some of the claims hold up to further testing, but they have not yet been reproduced by others.*
>
> *One exciting field is pro-host therapy, based on the theory that it's possible to take the natural immune system beyond its natural limits. If it works, it would make a stronger immune system, possibly preventing recurrences. This field is brand new, but the few technical papers I've seen are fascinating.*

It's true that as science learns more and more about herpesvirus, medicine is getting closer to being able to interfere with the virus's age-old strategies. It's also true that in the last ten years alone, our knowledge about this bothersome virus has increased exponentially. But progress may not continue at this rate. Fred Rapp, Ph.D., is Professor and Chairman of the Department of Microbiology at the Hershey Medical Center and American Cancer Society Professor of Virology: "We are doing some exciting work with understanding latency in herpesvirus. We've developed a cell-culture system which for the first time allows us to follow the virus as it goes in and out of latency—it's the first time *anyone's* been able to do that.

"Little pieces of information about herpesviruses are developed almost every day, but we are still missing some very critical epidemiological information about transmittability, contagiousness—some of the fundamental stuff we need to know if we are going to treat people. We are in an era where you can make fast progress, if you have the funds. But that's the problem here—funding. We have a disease that afflicts a lot of people, and very limited funds with which to conduct research."

The trend is not encouraging. Wendy J. Wertheimer, Director of Public Policy at the American Social Health Organization, charges that "the federal venereal disease prevention and control program will sustain an $8 million cut in funding in the fiscal year 1982. Of the total $3.7 billion budget of the National Institute of Health, the National Institute of Allergy and Infectious Disease will spend a mere $9 million on *all* sexually-transmitted diseases, and only $1.6 million on research on herpes." Dr. Rapp admits, "I don't believe that at the moment we have anything that will be a sure cure or for long-term use."

Of course, it's possible that science will find a herpesvirus vaccine that could be administered to the entire population to prevent infection in those who have not yet contracted the disease. The pharmaceutical giant Merck, Sharpe, and Dohme is now testing—in at least two separate programs—a vaccine that *may* be effective for inoculation of the general population against herpesvirus. Company officials warn, however, that such vaccines cannot help those *already* infected; who carry the virus particles in their nerve cells.

Don't worry about missing out on a possible herpes cure. When one is developed, it will make front-page headlines. Should a vaccine (or any other substance) be found to be effective against herpesvirus, it won't be kept a secret. Your doctor will know about it immediately.

Meanwhile, herpesvirus infections are better understood by perceiving the patient as a whole being, rather than as a statistic in a double-blind, placebo-controlled study. There are *proven* ways to help reduce the severity and frequency of herpesvirus attacks. The ideas in the next two chapters aren't quack cures, nor do we offer them as guaranteed, foolproof solutions. But they do present a number of common-sense approaches to what is obviously a physical *and* psychological problem.

12

Preventing the Spread of Herpes Simplex Virus

It's easier to keep out than get out. — MARK TWAIN

An ounce of prevention, Benjamin Franklin stated, is worth a pound of cure. And when no cure exists, Franklin's statement becomes even more to the point. Until biomedical science finds a way to cure herpesvirus infections, once you've acquired it, you must try to avoid two things:

1) transmitting the virus to uninfected persons, and

2) spreading the virus to uninfected parts of your body.

With some diseases, such as polio and measles, those who have caught the virus once make up the pool of non-susceptibles—those who can neither contract the disease nor spread it. With herpes simplex virus, unfortunately, a pool of non-susceptibles does not exist. Anyone who contracts herpesvirus leaves the pool of susceptibles and enters the pool of infectious persons, who are recurrently capable of spreading the disease. (About a third of those who do contract herpesvirus never get recurrences and are not considered infectious.) Therefore, simple prevention becomes the only way to combat the spread of this disease.

In the case of genital or oral herpesvirus, prevention is largely a simple matter of awareness.

Jessie W., a 25-year-old speech pathologist, lives in Philadelphia. For the past eight years, she has been dating the same boyfriend—who has had oral herpesvirus since childhood.

> Jessie: *I had been dating Joey for a couple of years. Of course, I noticed that occasionally he developed a cold sore on his upper lip. I didn't realize that it was contagious or anything more than the symptom of a cold. So I never avoided kissing him, and now I get a cold sore on my lip that's kind of like a mirror image of the site of Joey's cold sore.*
>
> Karen B.: *The doctor wanted to know who I got the herpes from. The truth is, I wasn't quite sure. I know a lot of guys, but I think I have a good idea who gave it to me. I don't see him any more. Once I noticed*

*something on him, but he told me not to worry about it, that it was just
a rash or something. I believed him.*

Herbert R.: *Years ago, I had a recurrence and I was with a woman who
wanted to make love. I wanted to too, so I didn't say anything: I wasn't
being devious; at the time, I thought I was being brave. I figured it might
hurt me a little, see, but for the sex it would be worth it. I didn't realize
the damn thing was contagious as hell.*

*Who knows how many women I've infected and who, in turn, in-
fected others? It's scary to think about. If only that doctor in Chicago
had known what the hell he was talking about! Now, I'm well aware of
the consequences of spreading it around. I'm sorry about infecting those
women—if I did. No one ever mentioned anything, you know. But it
was unintentional. . . .*

People with herpesvirus are plainly contagious when blisters or sores
are present. But virus particles have been successfully cultured from the
sites of outbreaks until the sore and its scab are completely healed and no
longer visible. To avoid spreading the infection, anyone with an active
herpesvirus infection must avoid physical contact with others. If someone
has genital sores, then obviously genital contact—no matter how slight or
brief—must be postponed until healing is complete. ("If I'm in the midst of a
recurrence," one sufferer told us, "then I won't get involved—at least not
with someone new.")

Question: *Don't only sexually promiscuous people contract the virus?*

Obviously not, since you can be infected with herpesvirus particles
from an inanimate object. It only takes one virion to cause an infection—and you don't have to be promiscuous to come in contact with a
single virus particle. On the other hand, those who are sexually active are
far more likely to be a source of herpesvirus infection. For example, Deirdre
O. is a prostitute who works Atlantic City's Pacific Avenue—the 42nd
Street of that resort city. She moved East with her sister, also a prostitute,
when the casinos opened. Tall, slender and well-built, Deirdre is extremely
popular.

Deidre: *Herpes? I know all about it, believe me! I get little infections all
the time, and all of them are curable, except the herpes. It really burns
when I'm with a john. But of course, mentioning it wouldn't be good for
business. Some people say it's not contagious, but I think it is. How else
did I get it? Occupational hazard, that's all. If it is contagious, I bet between my sister and me, we must've given it to a thousand guys. [She
laughs] But this sure isn't a convent down here, honey.*

Tina G. is 19. She's been a streetwalker on New York's West Side for
about two years.

Tina: *Yeah, I got it. Who doesn't? My old man says not to worry about
it, but I do. When I get the blisters, it hurts to work. I see sometimes*

four, five, six guys a day. When I get home, my old man knows only one question: "How much?" I can't afford to be sick. I asked the doc, "Can't you give me something?" but he said there's no cure, that he can't do anything for me. He doesn't know I'm working. I told him I got it from my boyfriend. Who knows, maybe I did. At first, whenever I got the blisters, I'd only French guys—but now I get the blisters in my mouth, too. They're like mouth ulcers, only they last longer and hurt more. But what am I supposed to do, quit working? My old man would just love that. . . .

JoAnne H., a 28-year-old prostitute from Philadelphia, has been in the business for four years. She doesn't walk the streets, but works for an "out-call massage service," meeting clients at their offices or hotels—even at their homes. Though she shares the prearranged fee with the massage parlor operators, she manages to take home as much as $1,200 a week, working five nights a week. JoAnne sees fifty to sixty men a month.

JoAnne: I've had every damn thing you can get—and it always seems like it's from the most respectable guys. The sleazy-looking types I wish I didn't have to be with are much cleaner. I've had syph twice, gonorrhea maybe four times, yeast and urinary tract infections a hundred times. But the real bitch is herpes. You can't get rid of it, ever. And it seems the more I work, the more it comes back.

The doctors act as if it's poison ivy. "Don't worry about it," they tell you. "It'll go away by itself. Don't work while it's acting up." Great advice, you know? With a herpes infection, it hurts like hell to screw—and then it gets worse. As it is, I lose five, sometimes six days a month because of my period. Some chicks don't mind—they just use their mouths then—but I like to be prepared for whatever the customer wants. I took some marketing classes in college, and one of the first laws of retail sales is "Never be sold out of any product." So when I'm not able to do everything, I don't work. But since I got herpes, I don't know where, I've been averaging another three or four days off a month.

Some chicks don't get it as often as I do, but they've all got it. One girl told me she thought she'd been rubbed raw; she thought that a guy had been, well, too big for her, you know. I took one look and said, "Sweetheart, that's herpes." She said, "No, it's not!" She didn't want it, so she didn't have it. Pretty smart!

My doctor told me there's nothing else of this God's earth that's more contagious than herpes during an infection. The rest of the time, it's not infectious—it lays quiet in the nerves, they say. That's why getting nervous and upset can set it off. I don't know if I've ever given it to a customer. No one's ever complained, and I have plenty of steadies. I may have given it to my husband, but he's not exactly Mister Innocent. He may have picked it up on his own. Was he angry? No, he likes the cash I make too much. As for me, it's not having herpes that bothers me, it's that it cuts into my work schedule.

Question: *I've heard that careful washing right after sex will prevent one from getting the virus.*

This is an excellent habit to develop, and *will* appreciably reduce the risk of contracting any sexually transmitted disease. But unfortunately, it's no guarantee against contracting herpesvirus. Once a virion has invaded your cells, no amount of scrubbing will forestall an infection.

Question: *Aren't condoms effective against the spread of herpesvirus?*

Unfortunately, no. Condoms have several possible flaws when it comes to preventing the transmission of viral particles. For one thing, if a woman is having a recurrence, her vaginal secretions are likely to be full of infectious herpesvirus. During intercourse, these secretions often spread across the entire genital area of both partners—including the man's testicles, abdomen, thighs, and buttocks.

If the *man* is afflicted with herpesvirus, condoms are still risky. Some experts claim that the tiny herpes simplex virion is small enough to penetrate the microscopic pores of most condoms. Dr. Lawrence Corey,head of the Virology Department of University of Washington's School of Medicine, has said, "we do know that under examination by the electron microscope, the diameter of the herpesvirus is smaller than the pores of the condom . . . and even when a condom is used properly, failures have been known to occur." Using a condom may reduce the odds against infection, but it should not encourage sex partners into thinking they are protected from spreading and contracting herpesvirus. Unfortunately, there is no sure way to prevent transferral of virions.

Acquiring a perspective of periodic infectiousness is 90 percent of the battle. Usually, a herpes virus patient is infectious only when sores are present. But as Debbie R. says, "I don't know whether I have lesions internally,out of sight. In terms of transmission and taking precautions to prevent transmission, that's a very uncomfortable thing to be aware of. I can never be sure that there isn't a lesion inside where I won't know about it."

One of the most disconcerting facts about herpesvirus that sufferers must accept is that there may be times when active viral particles can be cultured—in other words, when the individuals are contagious—without any sores or sensation being present at all. Carefully documented and well-controlled tests have demonstrated that virus particles may occasionally be present without any of the symptoms that usually accompany full-blown outbreaks. In answering a question along this line, *The Helper* replied:

> One investigator reported finding the presence of herpes simplex viruses in the urogenital tract of men who had no history of symptoms of genital herpes . . . the exact meaning with respect to infectiousness is not clear . . . herpes simplex viruses have been isolated from oral secre-

tions of persons between recurrences, though infectiousness has not been demonstrated.

"I feel I have a pretty good idea of when I'm infectious and when I'm not." Says Carrie E. "You take a chance in everything you do. Every time I pick up a fare, I take a chance of being robbed, raped, murdered, or worse. That's life. I hope I don't sound arrogant, but that's how I feel."

Further studies are underway to expand our understanding of this "silent shedding" of viral particles. But research indicated that silent shedders release about 10,000 times fewer virions than do patients in the midst of a recurrence. And only between 1 percent and 1½ percent of herpesvirus patients shed silently; anyone fearful of being in that rare group can be tested to disclose when herpesvirus are present on the skin's surface. In the overwhelming majority of cases, however, the familiar prodrome symptoms signal to the herpesvirus patient that a period of contagiousness has begun.

A *syndrome* is any group of symptoms that characterizes an abnormality or illness. A *prodrome* occurs *before* the onset of the syndrome—in other words, it is the first symptom before the main set of symptoms. As an example, the "symptoms" of a thunderstorm would be heavy rain, lightning, and thunder. The "prodrome" of a thunderstorm would be a darkening sky, and sounds of thunder in the distance.

Everyone who has experienced a herpesvirus prodrome describes his or her own personal set of signs and sensations, generally felt at the exact site of previous infections. The prodrome may vary from individual to individual, ranging from absolutely no warning at all (but fewer than 10% of all patients report no warning sensations) to rare cases of excruciating pain. The following are the most commonly described warning signals that may alert a herpesvirus patient to an impending outbreak:

• *Crawling:* the sensation that something is crawling or creeping beneath the surface of the skin. (*Herpes* is the Greek word that means "to creep;" *herpetology* is the study of snakes.)

• *Heat:* a warm, pulse-like throbbing at the site.

• *"Invisible scratch":* it feels as though there were a slight abrasion on the skin; yet none is visible.

• *Isolated sensations:* sometimes similar to the tingling or pins-and-needles feelings described below, but restricted to a different and seemingly inappropriate part of the body. One herpesvirus patient reports a sensation that occurs in her foot, but always precedes an outbreak in her genital region.

• *Itchiness:* The feeling that "something is there," on or just under the skin.

• *Malaise and general fatigue:* The general complaint of feeling "sick and tired" often signals an attack, but is non-specific. That is, no one part of the body feels bad; the patient simply feels poorly in general.

- *Muscular aches and pains:* Muscles near the nerve paths involved in the migration of virus particles sometimes ache or throb with a dull pain. In cases of oral herpesvirus, patients sometimes report that their cheeks and jaw muscles ache.
- *Neuralgia:* An impending viral attack is sometimes characterized by pain—usually mild, but sometimes quite sharp—radiating through the lower back or down the legs.
- *Phantom inflammation:* the area *feels* inflamed, and perhaps is even warm to the touch, yet is not visibly so.
- *Pins and needles:* as if a small patch of skin had "fallen asleep," much as a limb in a cramped position will lose sensation and then come back to life.
- *Poison-ivy itch:* the feeling that a dermatitis rash is about to develop.
- *Pressure:* the sensation that something is pushing under the skin, or pressing up against the surface. ("I feel something hard under the surface of the skin, like something is about to protrude. Sometimes, but not all of the time, it hurts.")
- *Prickly sensations:* like tiny jabs in the skin.
- *Slight surface achiness* on or near the site.
- *Swollen glands:* When an infection takes hold and the immune system is stimulated, the lymph glands swell. Although this symptom usually accompanies primary attacks of herpesvirus, many patients report swollen glands as a prodromal symptom. Perhaps the immune system anticipates the impending viral infection and begins to gear up against it, with increased activity in the lymph nodes.
- *Tingling:* an almost tickle-like feeling, sometimes as if there were a slight vibration beneath the skin.
- *Touch-sensitivity:* the skin feels sore, or as if a pimple were about to erupt.
- *Twitchiness:* as if there were a slight spasm or twitch beneath the skin.

What causes this wide range of sensations? The generally accepted theory is that the feelings common during the prodrome are caused by the virions' migration and the beginnings of their cellular invasion. We know that the nerves play a major role in viral migration, and the presence of herpesvirus "intruders" may disturb some of the communications of the nervous system. As the viral particles migrate from the ganglia toward the epidermal cells, they may irritate the nerves slightly and thereby create the sensations we call prodrome.

It's probable that the achy, throbbing discomfort is caused by the actual migration of the particles. Once the virions leave the safety of the nerve pathways, they begin invading cells beneath the skin surface. As these stricken cells swell, die, and disintegrate, they cause the itching and tingling that warn herpesvirus patients of an imminent outbreak.

Many people report having learned the art of recognizing prodrome feelings at the earliest possible moment, with practice and concentration. This ability is *the* most valuable asset in our arsenal against the spread of herpesvirus. Since recent laboratory tests have demonstrated that virus particles can be transmitted at the outset of prodrome sensations—before the actual development of any blisters—this alerts the herpesvirus patient that he or she has entered a period of transmittability. Infectious persons can then be especially careful to avoid physical contact with others and not to transfer virions to other parts of their own bodies—especially not the eyes, mouth, nose, or genitals; for if hygiene is not practiced, the disease can be spread to other parts of the body. Each new site of infection will then develop its own independent pattern of recurrence frequency, duration, and severity.

It is also crucial to keep sores from coming in direct or indirect contact with any object that can then result in a further infection. On May 14, 1982, writer Cristine Russell of the *Washington Post* Service reported on a study conducted at the University of California at Los Angeles. Researchers wanted to determine precisely how long a herpesvirus particle can survive outside the body. The study's results—which startled the medical world and will cause much rethinking of how some viral diseases are transmitted—were reported at a joint meeting of the American Pediatric Society and the Society for Pediatric Research in Washington, D.C.

> Dr. Trudy Larsen, a research fellow and pediatrician at UCLA . . . and her colleague Dr. Yvonne Bryson . . . took samples of herpes from patients' genital lesions and transmitted [the particles] to various surfaces. For even more realism, one genital herpes patient sat briefly on a toilet seat.
> They found that the virus survived on the toilet seat from 1½ to 4 hours. On a medical instrument . . . survival time increased to 18 hours. On cotton gauze . . . as long as 72 hours.

This study challenged the longstanding theory that herpesvirus can be transmitted only by direct physical contact and pointed up the hazards of sharing towels and clothing with persons suffering outbreaks of genital or oral herpesvirus.

Is preventing the spread of herpes simplex a tall order, then? Not really. If the occurence is oral, then kissing or sharing drinks, kitchen utensils, toothbrushes or cigarettes is *verboten*—but only temporarily.

Question: *I know I shouldn't kiss my children when I have an active herpesvirus cold sore on my lip. The older kids understand this, but my youngest one cries when I don't kiss her good night. What should I do?*

Most youngsters are able to understand the concept of contagiousness and deserve an explanation in simple, non-medical terms. Certainly you should explain that the "ban" on kissing is only temporary. One mother solved the problem by telling her offspring that the sore on her lip made it painful for her to kiss or be kissed—and so she asked for "a big hug" instead.

What about very young children for whom explanations won't suffice? Carroll Weinberg, M.D., Clinical Assistant Professor of Psychiatry and of Pediatrics at Philadelphia's Hahnemann Medical College, states that "a child should not have to depend solely on a parental kiss in order to feel loved. And though parents sometimes try to have their children feel wonderful all the time, the reality is that they cannot. In cases of oral herpes infection, there simply can be no kissing until the sore heals."

13

Easing Discomfort—
and Frequency—
of Recurrences

I get recurrences only three or four times a year. But I have a friend, a guy, who gets it every few weeks. That's tough to deal with. — DANIEL K.

Most herpesvirus sufferers agree that the first infection is by far the worst, accompanied by severe discomfort at the site of the lesions. Headaches, swollen glands, and shooting pains can also be present. Carrie E.'s infection was so severe that her physician almost hospitalized her.

> Carrie: *I couldn't imagine a worse experience. The pain in my groin was unbearable. I ran a high fever, had swollen glands, an unquenchable thirst, and a throbbing headache day and night. Urinating was excruciating, and I was drinking tremendous amounts of liquid because I was so thirsty.*
>
> Daniel K.: *My primary outbreak was pretty bad—lesions all over the shaft of my penis. Those first few days were terrible. At one point, the friction of my skin against my underwear was so painful that I couldn't even walk around.*
>
> *Then things started to heal up, but it must have been the better part of a month before it cleared up completely.*

Minor outbreaks and recurrences are usually accompanied by less pain. But each person reacts differently. Some persons with chronic infections experience almost no discomfort, while others with only mild recurrences—perhaps two or three small blisters—complain of being in agony.

Five basic symptoms are commonly reported during genital infections, usually occuring in combination:

1. *The pain of the sores themselves*—minor or severe—is an invariable symptom of a herpesvirus outbreak. Some patients dose themselves with narcotics, but the consensus among physicians is that these drugs fail to control the pain effectively. Codeine and its derivatives can often cause nausea and indirectly lead to constipation, making matters worse. So consult your doctor before trying *any* remedy. As the Centers for Disease Con-

trol in Atlanta advise, don't harm yourself with treatments that don't work—for you.

In her article, "Easing the Symptoms of HSV" (*The Helper*, March 1982), Carol Winter, B.S.N., recommends "two aspirin every three hours while awake, keeping the drug level constant to prevent peaks and valleys. Some patients report that topical anesthetics such as Xylocaine or Americane spray provide temporary relief, but [it] is limited." Aspirin substitutes (such as Tylenol) are also found to be effective.

Creams and ointments can delay healing and, as mentioned before, may actually help the virus spread to uninfected tissue nearby. Most patients find that the best way to promote healing is to keep the lesions dry and clean. Some doctors advise soaking the sores (sitz bathing), provided that such treatments last no more than ten minutes. Patients sit in tubs into which Epsom salts, Burrow's Solution, or other drying agents have been added.

In his excellent book *Herpes: Cause and Control*, William H. Wickett, Jr., M.D., recommends the use of Burrow's Solution applied in cool compresses two or three times a day. Dr. Wickett also believes that Milk of Magnesia can relieve pain: "Do not shake the bottle, but allow it to sit on the shelf for several days. Then pour off the liquid on the top. Using a long cotton swab, obtain some of the thick material at the bottom of the bottle. Daub that on sores."

Afterwards, never dry the sores by rubbing them with a towel; any friction delays healing. Pat dry with disposable bathroom tissue, or better yet, use a hair dryer with the temperature set to low. During healing periods, loose clothing is advisable; cotton is best.

2. *Itching:* During prodrome and the actual outbreak, aspirin and aspirin substitutes may effectively reduce itching. Some patients report that applying icepacks decreases the itching (and in some cases, even prevents outbreaks when applied early in the prodrome). Ms. Winter advises women with vaginal itching to check with their doctors to rule out concurrent vaginitis.

3. *Burning upon urination (dysuria)* affects men only if they suffer from lesions in the urethra or at the very tip of the glans penis. But it is a common problem in women, who experience pain whenever uric acid—the chemical that causes the burning sensation—comes in contact with the open lesions. "I always cover any sores with Vaseline before I urinate," says Emma D., a 38-year-old computer programmer from Phoenix. "It really works for me. But Vaseline slows the healing process, so I carefully wash it off afterwards."

Many doctors advise patients to urinate while in a bathtub of water to ease the sting of the uric acid. Patient can also dilute the urine *internally*, by drinking plenty of fluids.

"Some people find pouring hydrogen peroxide or water over the perineum [the area between the anus and the external genitalia] while voiding is quite soothing," writes Carol Winter. She adds that should the dysuria persist, it is important to have a clinician check for bacterial infection.

4. *Heavy vaginal discharge* is an uncomfortable symptom frequently present in primary infections, making it more difficult to keep the afflicted area clean and dry. Care should be taken to control the discharge. Some women wear minipads in their underwear. Others prefer tampons, but tampons can irritate open lesions and if used, should be inserted carefully and changed frequently. If careful hygiene is not practiced, constant touching of the infected areas could lead to further spread of the virus particles.

5. *Fatigue:* Illnesses—including herpesvirus infections—tax the body. The solution is as much rest as is practically possible. Though it may be difficult to take a day or two off from work or school, it's better than getting run down and becoming subject to lengthy and severe recurrences.

You may be eligible for compensation for time you may have missed from work due to herpesvirus outbreaks. But due to embarassment or ignorance, some herpesvirus patients are reluctant to file a claim under their company (or their own) health insurance plans. Leon Adoni, M.D., a respected dermatologist in Elkins Park, Pennsylvania, addresses this problem by saying: "Herpesvirus is an important medical condition that should not be ignored. A definite diagnosis should be made. Many medical plans cover problems such as acne—and if a plan will cover acne, it will cover herpes infections!"

Particularly in women, the symptoms and discomfort of a primary outbreak can often be so severe that patients are unable to go to work. People incapacitated by herpesvirus infections should take advantage of their employers' health plan or sick-leave program. Any health care worker, dental hygienist, nurse, or doctor who contracts herpesvirus on the job is eligible to recover any loss of wages and medical expenses through Worker's Compensation insurance. If necessary, those patients should have their family doctors document the illness with a letter or report.

Some Dos and Don'ts

• *Do* be alert for the prodrome symptoms, which warn of an upcoming herpesvirus outbreak. In most cases, your period of contagiousness begins then.

• *Do* apply ice or an icepack to the sites of previous infections when you first notice the prodrome. Though this technique doesn't guarantee that an outbreak won't materialize, many herpesvirus patients suggest that outbreaks "chilled" at the onset are less painful, less severe, and less long-lasting. Viral particles replicate best at body temperature, so local application of cold may well aid in reducing the herpesvirus's symptoms and severity. But be careful not to overdo things and damage your skin by prolonged exposure to freezing temperatures.

• *Don't* ever intentionally break open a blister. The fluid in each vesicle could contain millions of infectious virions. Releasing these herpesvirus particles just permits them to infect nearby cells. Breaking a blister also opens the door for secondary infections, which only prolong healing. Herpesvirus lesions that heal on their own do not normally scar, while blisters broken prematurely may leave scars.

• *Do* practice strict hygiene during recurrences. Many people unconsciously touch their oral or genital sores while asleep. During outbreaks, therefore, it's good to develop the habit of washing your hands with a mild detergent soap upon arising—especially before rubbing the "sleep" out of your eyes.

Remember that recent studies have shown that virus particles can survive for as long as seventy hours on cotton gauze—a material that shares many of the characteristics of towels, washcloths, and light clothing. During periods of infectiousness, keep all towels, toothbrushes, and other potentially "sharable" objects away from others, particularly children.

• *Don't* pick or scratch at sores. Just as with poison ivy or acne, disturbing the sore only increases the time required for complete healing.

• *Do* keep the area around the outbreak clean and dry—probably the best ways to speed the healing process.

• *Do* consider adding a drying agent to your bathing water. Many doctors recommend Epsom salts and certain other drying agents, but results vary widely. Some people prefer warm water for bathing, others cool or lukewarm. Consult your physician, but remain alert to your body's reaction to whatever may be prescribed and use what works best for you.

Helping Prevent Recurrences

Since the herpesvirus cannot be destroyed as long as it lies dormant, the best way to keep it under control is to prevent it from migrating back to the skin surface. Most of the time, after all, herpesvirus gets along fine inside the nervous system—which is why it is allowed to remain there. The trick is discovering what makes it "want" to leave the safety and security of the ganglia—and then deprive the virus of that stimulus, to keep it from getting restless in the first place.

Herpesvirus patients and their doctors have long observed that certain activities seem to precede outbreaks. In *Herpes: Cause and Control*, Dr. Wickett describes ten "triggers" which he believes can cause a fresh outbreak of herpesvirus infection:

Athletics and excessive, strenous physical activity can trigger recurrences.

Change of seasons—particularly spring to summer and summer to fall—seems to stimulate many oral herpes simplex infections.

Diseases, particularly serious ones, tax the immune system and permit latent herpesvirus to create new infections.

Foods containing high levels of argenine "have been indicated as possible culprits. Nuts, seeds, and onions are a few . . . that seem to be active in reducing our resistance to the disease," reports Dr. Wickett. Herpes folklore holds that eating chocolate and nuts can cause recurrences, but there has been no substantiation of this. Chocolate and nuts *can* cause allergies and acne, and both are high in an amino acid known as argenine, which was once believed to encourage the growth of herpesvirus particles. But we have found no test results that confirm that eating argenine-rich foods contributes to recurrences.

Menstrual periods: Dr. Wickett suggests that the considerable hormonal changes that occur in a woman's body just before menstruation may be why some women report a pattern of recurrences just prior to their period; but the overwhelming majority of women do not find this to be the case.

Sexual activity, it is suggested, can have an emotional and physiological impact on some people that is intense enough to cause a herpesvirus recurrence.

Smoking, according to Dr. Wickett, causes a marked drop in the immune response—hence making outbreaks more likely.

Trauma, or damage to skin tissue, has been known to provoke herpesvirus recurrences at the site of the injury.

Ultraviolet radiation: sunlight is known to initiate outbreaks of herpesvirus sores, especially on the lips of those who spend a lot of time in the sun—or at the beginning of the outdoor season.

But "of all the indirect factors in herpes flareups," writes Dr. Wickett, "stress is by far the most significant." How you behave in the presence of stress—how you react to, anticipate, cope with, and avoid it—has a great impact on your immune system and, therefore, on your ability to keep recurrent infections at bay.

The Physiology of Stress

The concept of stress evolved in the science of physics, where the word "stress" is used to describe a force that has the measurable ability to affect a physical object. Dr. Hans Selye, a pioneer in the field, views stress as "the non-specific response of the body to any demand upon it." Dr. Selye describes the General Adaptation Syndrome, or GAS—a system of reaction consisting of three stages.

First is the "alarm state"—an intricate physiological response that increases the body's ability to react quickly and exert itself physically in an emergency. In the case of a child darting in front of your car, of course, flight—steering away—is not possible and wouldn't stop you from running down the child. "Fight"—that is, trying to bring the car to a screeching halt—is the appropriate way to avoid the accident. The average driver reacts in a split second. Even before you could think to jam on the brakes, the alarm stage is under way, involving many cooperating bodily functions.

During the alarm stage, the hypothalamus, a part of your brain stem, activates the pituitary gland, which in turn releases a hormone (ACTH) into the bloodstream. When this hormone reaches the adrenal glands located atop the kidneys, it stimulates them to release adrenaline and cortisone, which in turn help direct blood from various internal organs to the brain and muscles.

Next, is the "resistance stage," in which the body begins reacting to the stressful stimulus by coordinating its musculature for swift, efficient action. Accompanying this reflexive action are the *emotional* aspects of stress—fear and anger. Hearing becomes more acute, eyesight sharpens as the pupils dilate and become more sensitive to light. Blood pressure rises, speeding other hormones throughout the body. Breathing becomes shallow and rapid, increasing the intake of oxygen. The spleen releases red blood cells that rush oxygen to organs of the body that are under pressure to perform.

All this happens in seconds. As soon as the emergency is over, adrenalin and other hormones are still being pumped through the bloodstream; the system is still stimulated from its original alarm reaction. Eventually, though, the body begins to return to a normal state. The various systems calm down, and the body continues in its regular fashion.

But what *is* its regular fashion? If small children darted out in front of your car all day long, how would your body react? Time and again, it would mobilize itself for action, of course; but these intense reactions would swiftly deplete your energy, to say nothing of your ability to handle such emergencies in a competent manner. This repeated "alarm" stimulation results in Selye's third stage: exhaustion. People who constantly perceive stresses (and therefore, who react more frequently) are likely to become "stress-exhausted." And when this kind of bodily depletion occurs too frequently, stress becomes a proven immunosuppressor, lowering the body's resistance and leaving it vulnerable to a wide range of diseases and infections.

Cortisone is one of the many substances secreted into the blood during times of stress, and microbiologists have found that in laboratory animals at least, viruses are much more devastating when injected together with varying quantities of cortisone. Dr. Paul J. Rosch, president of the American Institute of Stress in Yonkers, N.Y., claims that some conditions of emotional stress can suppress the production of interferon, the body's natural antiviral agent. In addition, stress in general retards the body's ability to produce the antibodies it needs to fight all types of infections.

Stress Versus Health

Doctors are discovering that more and more diseases are at least partly psychosomatic in origin. For example, hypertension, or high blood pressure, which causes strokes, heart disease, and kidney damage, is at times directly attributable to stress. Surgeons and firemen, whose jobs are extremely stressful, have a high incidence of hypertension in their ranks.

Arteriosclerosis is a condition whereby fatty substances are deposited in the arteries. Excess adrenaline is now known to contribute to the buildup of cholesterol in the cardiovascular system. Accordingly, the arteries are narrowed and when the coronary arteries are affected, then less blood reaches the heart muscle, which is deprived of needed oxygen. Studies of race car drivers have demonstrated that stress causes the triglyceride levels in the blood to rise dramatically: for as long as three hours after a race, the drivers' tryglyceride levels were still 200 percent above normal—and this condition is thought to contribute to arteriosclerosis.

Peptic ulcer is the condition most popularly associated with stress. The stomach uses hydrocloric acid to help break down foods during digestion—but it also secretes hydrocloric acid during moments of duress and emotional upset. And when no food is present for the acid to act upon, it can literally digest the stomach lining, creating the familiar ailment of the hard-driven businessman.

Robert L. Woolfolk, Ph.D. and Frank G. Richardson, Ph.D. are the authors of *Sanity and Survival* (Sovereign Books, 1978). "Even if one is very conservative in evaluating the available evidence," they write, "the list of physical maladies in which stress probably plays a role is quite long. Migraine headaches, backaches, asthma, arthritis, and even cancer have been linked to stress . . . But the detrimental effect of stress upon body tissue is only a part of the story . . . our environment and the view we take of it is central to many psychological and psychiatric problems as well."

Richard Hamilton, M.D., author of *The Herpes Book*, writes that "Stress, more than any other factor, demonstrates the triparte relationship between our feelings, our behavior, and the functioning of our natural defense mechanisms. Stress is so compellingly linked with lowered resistance to disease and decreased immune system activity that doctors have begun to regard it as having some predictive value in human illness . . . My experience with hundreds of herpes patients has demonstrated that stress is cited more often than anything else as a correlate with repeated and frequent recurrences."

Stress and Herpesvirus

Many people we interviewed reported fresh outbreaks when they were getting anxious over final exams, romantic difficulties, or financial troubles. Bill S. is a 34-year-old carpenter who, by his own definition, leads a hectic life. He contracted genital herpesvirus six years ago and suffers frequent recurrences—about ten a year.

> Bill: *I'm a nervous individual, and I get outbreaks almost every month. My doctor told me that being upset and hyper all the time can trigger it. But I can't help it. I got three kids at home, and with this economy, if I go out of business, I lose it all. So I got a right to be nervous.*
>
> *I bid on big jobs and work under contractors. We have tough schedules to meet, with no flexibility. The bottom line is to have the job finished on time, and on budget. But sometimes things that aren't my fault screw up the job. Like if material don't arrive on time, that makes me nervous. I got bills to pay, employees to pay, and if a job goes wrong, it's my reputation. When a job is almost finished and I hear we won't be getting lumber when they said that we would—well, I really get upset. And almost every time, I get that itchy feeling, and a day or two later, I got the blisters again. Sometimes it's so predictable I could set my watch by it. I know I got to work on the nervousness bit. But in this business, I don't have much control, you know?*

Marie Y., a second-year law student in New Orleans, is 24 and has had genital herpesvirus for four years. She found that her recurrences have a definite correlation to stressful situations.

> Marie: *My primary outbreak was a nasty one, but I didn't have another outbreak for more than a year. Then I was cramming for the LSATs. I have a history of not doing well on those standardized tests, and I was anxious as hell about the exam. So I stayed up all night for about a week and really got myself run down.*
>
> *I hadn't had sex, but I had a recurrence. It wasn't half as bad as my first time, but it hurt a lot to urinate. The glands around my pelvic area were slightly swollen, and I felt fatigued. I don't know if it was the stress alone, or the fact that I was run down—probably the combination gave the herpes the go-ahead to attack.*
>
> *It's interesting, but some of my female friends who have herpes say that intense sex—lots of it, for a long time—causes them to have outbreaks. Not me. I can have a marathon weekend and not even get a tingle. But when finals come around, or when I have to brief a difficult case for moot court, I can just about count on getting a recurrence. I get nervous easily; I'm paranoid about speaking in public—not very good for a lawyer, right?—and prepping for moot court gives me a lot of anxiety. I can feel myself getting "amped up," and sure enough, about two*

or three days later, bingo! I get an outbreak.

Daniel K.: *Being nervous and tense can cause an outbreak—I'd heard that in the support group, but I've actually seen it in my own life. I had two cats, both of them since I was a kid. I had been quite attached to them, and they were closer to me than most people are. Two years ago, they both died within a couple of months of each other. I couldn't have been more upset if they were people, and I proceeded to have my worst outbreak since the primary infection. Looking back, I realize that the death of the cats was the most upsetting thing that has happened to me in the last five years or so, and the outbreak was no mere coincidence.*

It's clear that persons who are subjected to stressful situations and lifestyles suffer more recurrences. The reason is not clear, though some theories suggest that stress *itself* may stimulate dormant virions into sudden activity. But the important point is that people who take it easy suffer fewer recurrent herpesvirus attacks.

What exactly can you do to minimize your "alarm" response? There are a variety of different techniques, as we'll see in the next chapter.

14

The Psychology of Stress

> *There is no illness of the body apart from the mind.* — SOCRATES

A *stressor* is defined as anything—internal or external—that subjects you to psychological or physical arousal. Waiting in a traffic jam, breathing polluted air, arguing with a friend, getting fired from a job (or merely *worrying* about getting fired) can all be stressful—but each stressor can also be perceived on different levels. And sometimes the stress may not be so obvious. For example, herpesvirus patients experience more than average fear and anxiety in their dealings with the uninfected world. Telling a prospective sex partner that you carry herpesvirus (even with the advice given in Chapter 6) is not exactly easy, nor something to which you'd look forward. Wondering whether an "uninformed" lover will contract the disease is also stressful. Some individuals contract herpes simplex outside of marriage and do not want to infect their spouses—but find intolerable the thought of "admitting" what seems like proof of adultery.

In day-to-day interaction, everything may seem to be cordial and relatively pleasant. Yet these troubled individuals may feel fatigue, anger easily, catch cold more easily than normal, have trouble getting a good night's sleep. What's happening is that chronic unconscious fears cause a subtle, but quite real alarm stage. These hidden stressors then cause the body to run through the General Adaptation Syndrome over and over again.

What you eat and drink has a marked effect on how you handle stress. Caffeine is a notorious stimulant, and a nervous system revved up with too much tea or coffee will tend to overreact to ordinary stimuli. On the other hand, many stress-harried individual try to dampen their nervous systems' reactions by dosing themselves with pills and alcohol. These depressants do reduce stress temporarily, by making stimuli less noticeable. But they take their own toll on the system: the misery of a hangover is almost impossible to cure, except by the passage of time.

On a broader scale, stess reactions tend to use up the body's supply of a number of nutrients (particularly the B-complex vitamins). And because of poor nutrition, some of the nutrients may not be replaced. For a full discussion of the inverse relationship between herpesvirus infections and good nutrition, see the next chapter.

Sleep, together with adequate waking rest, helps any herpesvirus patient handle stress more effectively. Most of us need between six and eight hours of sleep a night. If the sleep period is interrupted, or if there is simply not enough of it, the natural Rapid Eye Movement (REM) dream cycles do not occur. For reasons not wholly understood, it's dreaming—not mere sleep itself—that seems to refresh the mind. An individual who's missed out on his REM cycles will awaken "on the wrong side of the bed," displaying signs of anxiety, distraction, irritability, depression and poor concentration. Moreover, fatigue caused by insufficient sleep puts a strain on all bodily systems, robbing the immune system of the energy it needs to ward off recurrent herpesvirus infections.

If you are willing to take an *active* role in managing stress, there's a great deal you can do. In her article in *New York* Magazine, "Stress Can Be Good For You," Susan Seliger writes that "A person who feels in control of his life can channel stressful energy and make himself healthier than those who avoid conflict altogether. Researchers are finding that bad stress is triggered by the feeling that one's decisions are useless, that life is overwhelming and beyond personal control." In a nutshell, stress can best be managed by anticipating the unavoidable events that are bound to cause it, and by mentally rehearsing and preparing for them. In a study of 259 executives, Suzanne Kobasa, Ph.D., "found that certain people seemed able to handle stress no matter how intense their job pressures; if people felt a sense of purpose, viewed change as a challenge and not a threat, and believed they were in control of their lives, they were not adversely affected by stress."

Though most stresses do arise from external stimuli, their degree of effect depends upon the psychological "reception" they meet in your personal psyche. For our purposes, stress can be considered an *internal* force, not an external one. The most important factor in understanding stress is that it's largely subjective: *an individual's perception of an event is the prime determinant of how stressful it is.* William Shakespeare could have been thinking about stress management when he had Hamlet say, "There is nothing good or bad but thinking makes it so."

Knowing about the dynamics of stress and its effect on you can help reduce it—often significantly. The stresses you face may be unavoidable, but the ways you find to deal with them are entirely up to you! For stress reaction is *learned* behavior. And what you have learned, you can unlearn; or at least modify.

In his book, *The Relaxation Response*, Herbert Benson, M.D., defines emotional stress as an environmental demand that requires behavioral adjustment. You can learn to resist your body's stress reactions, in exactly the way you would politely resist a pushy, obnoxious, overbearing salesman—by refusing to go along, and detaching yourself from them. For example, you should consider anger—which can cause a clinically observable stress reaction—as a form of hangover. While a mugger has a revolver to your head, you feel nothing but fear. Later, at the police station, is when you may feel anger—because the immediate threat has been removed.

Anger, then, is the *after-effect* of a stressful event. It's the frustrated sense of having been wronged. On the other hand, anxiety (or as most people know it, worry) is an emotion of *anticipation* or expectation. It's the feeling of helplessness that occurs *before* an event you're convinced will be stressful. Usually, the basis of your anxiety will prove unfounded, but the damage has already been done—your system has been geared up as if for a real-life event. Even when your greatest fear *is* realized (failing an important exam, for example), the attention and mental energy that went into worrying has no effect upon the outcome, except possibly to make things worse ("I was so worried about the exam I couldn't study").

The trick here is a kind of inner assertiveness training. Start by understanding that you *don't* have to react automatically, like a pre-programmed robot, to whatever life throws your way. By being more aware of your own characteristic reactions to a stressful situation, you can significantly reduce the negative energy-wasting reactions that do nothing to resolve the problem. Anticipating this kind of *regular* stress is not only beneficial in itself, but people who make a habit of it seem to handle stress more effectively.

"Recognizing that stress is a factor in recurrence," Dr. Luby writes, "can recurrences be prevented by stress management? Can techniques such as biofeedback or relaxation therapy perhaps influence . . . immunologic systems?"

Sam Knox: "We don't believe that stress management or meditation will make the herpes go away, but these methods do help individuals learn to accept and deal with herpesvirus—just like arthritis, for example. Though the physical problem will still exist, you can relieve the burden of the psychological problem, which may aggravate the physical condition." But according to Ted A. Grossbart, Ph.D., of the Department of Psychology at the Beth Israel Hospital, Harvard Medical School, hypnosis is "one of the most effective stress-reduction techniques." He points out that fifty-four years ago, the University of Vienna's Dr. Robert Heilig and Dr. Hans Hoff used hypnotic techniques not only to alleviate but experimentally to produce oral herpes outbreaks. And "in 1981, Dr. R. Arone di Bertolino of the University of Bologna reported hypnotic treatment of nine patients with weekly or bimonthly genital herpes recurrence. A year and a half after treatment, six people had not had any recurrences and three had experienced only one or two recurrences yearly. My own research also suggests that, while no panacea, a range of hypnotic, imaging and psychotherapeutic techniques is well worth further investigation."

> Marie Y.: *My roommate has herpes, and ever since she learned this relaxation exercise from her psychologist, she swears she's been able to keep the herpes from recurring—but only when she gets the tingling sensations first. Apparently, that gives her enough time to psyche herself out of the infection. She does this meditation thing: quiet, eyes closed, relaxing all of her muscles. I guess it works. Finals are coming up for this semester. Maybe I should try it.*

In Appendix C, "Suggested Further Reading," we mention several important books that offer readers a variety of ways to reduce stress, including meditation and relaxation exercises. For example, *Life After Stress* by Martin Shaffer, Ph.D., discusses six modes of relaxation techniques: deep-breathing exercises, deep-muscle relaxation, meditation, stretching exercises (including yoga), biofeedback, and a form of self-hypnosis known as autogenic training. It's not a question of which is more effective; rather, which fit best with your lifestyle and personality. Relaxation techniques, if used correctly, can reduce the quantity and the extent of everyday stress reactions.

Such periods of *deliberate* relaxation do more than just prepare you to face life's next assortment of slings and arrows. There are definite physical effects: your breathing slows, becoming deeper and fuller. The heart slows too, beating in a more even and rhythmic manner. Muscles throughout the body relax. Brain waves change, as thought become more "loose" and free associative; accumulated tensions and resentments seem to fade away. Most conscious relaxers report immediate improvement in their outlook on life. And with mental *and* physical energy levels on the rebound, they feel "recharged." Remember, by decreasing your stress level, you raise your resistance and immune system activity.

In addition, as Dr. Luby points out, some patients report that they have invented their own techniques for reducing stress and preventing recurrences.

> Diane K.: *Sometimes I get a tingling feeling, or what I think is a tingling sensation, in my vagina during sex. I don't know if that's what they call the prodrome, but if I'm worried I might be causing a recurrence, I've got a motto about stopping sex: "When in doubt, take it out." So, if I'm having sex and it starts to feel strange, I stop. No one's ever gotten mad about having to stop; it hasn't happened that much anyway.*

Kim B. is a 26-year-old housewife living in Los Angeles. She has had oral herpes virus for six years, but believes that she can "will" away outbreaks as soon as she feels the prodrome sensations.

> Kim: *I've noticed that if I start to worry about it or try to treat it, like with Camphophenique or Kanka or other things that are supposed to get rid of it, it usually erupts into a full-blown sore. But when I don't fuss with it or pick at it like I used to, it usually goes away. It doesn't seem logical, but basically, I say to myself, "Okay now, I am not going to get a cold sore. I'm not going to touch it. It will not erupt. It will go away." The first time I tried that, I wasn't sure it would work. But it did work. Ever since then, I've done the same thing, and it always kept the sore from erupting. The only time my procedure failed was when I went on vacation to Florida with two girlfriends. There was a lot of sun, and I know that can trigger an outbreak. All three of us got them on our lips—and no, we weren't kissing!*

Dr. Paul J. Rosch explains how this "mind over lesions" technique may be possible: "There is evidence that on the cell walls of lymphocytes are receptor sites for ACTH, the prime hormone released under stress, and other brain hormones. This implies that the brain can 'talk' directly to the immune system. People may be able to tune into that 'conversation' and even influence it, just as they can be trained to influence pulse rate and skin temperature through biofeedback. People may have the ability to cure themselves."

In short, then:

- *Don't* let stress and the pressures of daily life debilitate you. This can only mean more frequent, prolonged, and severe recurrences. Learn some relaxation techniques to let off the pent-up steam and hostilities we all build up. Avoid or modify behavior that leads to stress and tension at home, or on the job.
- *Don't* panic when you experience a recurrence. Fear is an extreme form of stress and actually reduces your immune system's ability to defend your body against infection. Panic ("high-speed worry") merely slows your physiological and emotional recovery.
- *Don't* feel guilty about recurrences. Think of genital sores as simple cold sores. Or employ a technique many psychologists recommend: imagine that the sores are the result of an allergy—to asparagus, say. In a very real way, you *are* allergic to herpesvirus particles. Some people are immune to them, never developing herpes simplex lesions, no matter how often they are exposed. Others, unfortunately, are susceptible. Of course, you shouldn't forget that the cause is contagious, but comparing the lesions to an allergy often helps you gain a more balanced perspective.

THE PSYCHOLOGY OF STRESS

15

A Second Look at the Immune System

Sometimes I have a recurrence without prodrome and sometimes I feel the prodrome and nothing happens. — DEBBIE R.

Just as clouds do not necessarily mean that it will rain, prodromal symptoms do not guarantee a herpesvirus outbreak. Some patients, like Debbie, report feeling the prodrome symptoms—only to be happily surprised when no outbreak develops.

How can the prodrome occur without having an attack materialize? When viral particles migrate to the site of previous infections, whether they succeed in creating a new sore depends on a variety of circumstances. If the particles that have migrated to the skin surface are not virulent or numerous enough to establish themselves, then a new infection will not occur. In other instances, the herpesvirus particles are able to launch a cellular invasion, but the immune system is in top form, preventing the virus from getting a significant foothold.

Although the immune system may not *seem* very effective to someone troubled by recurrent infections of herpesvirus, it actually does a very commendable job. If it was not effective against the very first herpesvirus, the very first infection would be fatal. To help minimize the severity of recurrences, it's important to understand a bit more about how the immune system operates.

Throughout history, physicians noticed that patients seemed incapable of contracting certain diseases more than once. Could exposure to an infection confer some kind of immunity to it? To protect individuals from the smallpox epidemics that used to ravage the Orient, 15th century Chinese medical practitioners encouraged them to inhale the powdered scabs of smallpox sores. The technique was usually effective—but only if the patient survived the treatment.

In old England, the sores of any disease were referred to as "pox" or "pocks"—a term that survives in today's word, "pockmark." Syphilis produces huge sores in its tertiary stage, and so was termed "the great pox."

The smaller blisters of a then-widespread viral infection were called the "small pox," by contrast. The 18th century English physician Edward Jenner noticed that milkmaids who had been infected with the rarely fatal cowpox disease never seemed to contract the more often deadly smallpox. He concluded that whatever the body did to prevent reinfection of cowpox also served to block infection by smallpox. And in 1796, Jenner created history's first successful immunization.

A century later, Louis Pasteur injected weakened cholera bacteria into chickens, trusting that because the bacteria were too weak to assert themselves, the birds would not develop the disease. He hoped that the birds' immune systems, in striking out against the mild infection, would develop the ability to handle full-strength cholera germs. Weeks later, Pasteur injected the same chickens with strong, unimpaired cholera bacteria. To his delight, the birds did not sicken. The infection never materialized, proving Pasteur's theory of acquired immunity to be true. But until the science of immunology came into being, it was still not clear exactly *how* this immunity was acquired.

Immunology, simply, is the branch of medicine that studies the body's ability to discover, identify, control, and dispose of substances foreign to it—whether they be dead or alive, organic or inorganic, visible or microscopic. Earlier in the 20th century, two different theories of immunity began to gain acceptance. The *cellular theory* advanced the idea that certain cells in the bloodstream acted as soldiers—that is, scouted around for foreign matter and upon finding it, destroyed it. The *humoral theory* of immunity held that some cells could produce and secrete into the bloodstream chemicals that deterred an infection from progressing.

We now know that both theories are correct. The immune system is not only able to find and dispose of foreign bodies, it can also identify and fight a single, specific invader while ignoring other substances. Anything that intrudes into the body and threatens to cause an infection is called an *antigen.* Under normal circumstances, the presence of any antigen causes the immune system to design a specific protein—or antibody—to respond to the particlar configuration of protein molecules on that antigen's surface. These molecular configurations are called *determinants*, which "mark" the antigens and thereby alert the antibodies to attack them. Determinants, usually found only on foreign molecules, sometimes appear on the surface of normal cells that have been invaded by infectious organisms.

Either way, these determinants signal circulating antibodies to bind themselves to the antigens. And most importantly, antibodies can remember what a particular antigen "looks" like for future reference, should that bacteria or virus ever enter the body again. We know now that smallpox and cowpox are caused by two closely related viruses. The cowpox virus is not identical to the smallpox virus, but because their surface molecular configurations are so similar, cowpox antibodies will also bind themselves to smallpox determinants. This process of *agglutination* hand-cuffs the antigens in a sense, restricting their movement and incapacitating them in other ways. (Movie fans will recall the scene in *Fantastic Voyage* in which Raquel Welch was attacked by antibodies in her "host's" bloodstream.) Then, held in place by a clump of antibodies, the antigens are quickly devoured by T-cells, transported from the site, and eventually eliminated through the kidneys.

With regard to intruders, the immune system's memory often lasts for the life of the organism. And so vaccination hopes to stimulate the immune system into creating lasting antibodies to fight specific diseases the body has not yet contracted. (The word comes from the Latin word *vacca*, for cow, the animal of Jenner's observations.) Vaccinations are used regularly to produce immunity against various viruses and bacteria, including typhoid, smallpox, whooping cough, hepatitis B, rabies, mumps, cholera, diptheria, polio, tetanus, and yellow fever. But in all vaccines, the basic principle is the same: killed or weakened viruses are injected into the patient or ad-ministered orally. (In most vaccines, the viruses have been treated chemically so that they are unable to replicate effectively. In "live" vac-cines, small doses of disease-causing virions are administered; and some ex-tremely dangerous side effects have been observed.) As the disabled par-ticles circulate throughout the body, the immune system never "realizes" that these invaders are essentially harmless; upon recognizing potential threats to the body, the immune system shoots first and asks questions later. (And indeed, many vaccinated people do experience a "reaction," with slight fever, lassitude, and acheyness—the symptoms of a very low-grade viral infection.) The immune system resists these new antigens by creating antibodies that will remain in the system long after these first virus particles are overcome—and provide protection against future infections of the same virus.

Vaccines are not effective against all viral diseases, though. For exam-ple, the common cold is caused by an enormous number of unrelated viruses, and a vaccine can work only against specific or closely related virions. But both the antibodies and the immune system's "memory" re-main alert to those particular antigens forever (though an occasional booster shot is sometimes administered just to make sure that the immune system hasn't "forgotten"). Should those same specific antigens ever appear again, antibodies already present in the body will mount a "pre-emptive strike," preventing the new infection from making any progress at all.

In a sense, then, a primary herpes infection "vaccinates" you against later recurrences. The first attack is usually more severe because during the initial infection, your immune system is at a disadvantage, not being prepared with antibodies to attack those specific herpesvirus particles. Days pass before your body is able to manufacture the right antibodies. But during a later recurrence, the appropriate antibodies are able to keep the infection in check at the site of the outbreak. If the immune system is successful—and in the case of healthy individuals, it usually is—the body soon returns to its previous state of health and activity.

In addition to protecting the body from repeated infections, the immune system has other important functions in maintaining the health of an individual. After a viral attack, for example, when the body is littered with dead and dying cells, the immune system is charged with marshalling and removing cell "corpses" so that they can be eliminated from the body. But there are times when the immune system behaves *too* efficiently in its efforts to destroy invaders. This overreaction can result in allergies and hypersensitivities to normally harmless substances. In rare cases, the immune system may go awry and mount a response to some of the body's own cells, as in certain forms of arthritis. One serious disease suspected to result from this process of auto-immunity is multiple sclerosis. A more common instance of this auto-immune error occurs during rheumatic fever. Originally, the immune system mounts an attack against invading streptococcal bacteria in the patient's throat—a perfectly normal reaction to "strep" bacteria. But the antigenic determinants of the streptococcus bear an unfortunate similarity to the surfaces of certain cells in joint tissue and heart muscle—and this mistaken identity fools the antibodies into attaching themselves to body tissue, often inflicting severe damage in the process.

To the ever-watchful lymphocytes, any foreign molecule is an invader. And so the immune system also fails to differentiate between a lethal viral particle and a life-saving transplanted organ. If the patient's system is functioning optimally, it will automatically reject the new tissue because it contains foreign substances—antigens—resulting in the death of the new organ. Therefore, when doctors prepare a patient for an organ transplant, they try to diminish the body's tendency to attack foreign matter by *immunosuppression*—administering different chemotherapies that greatly decrease the ability of the patient's cells to reproduce. Without fairly rapid cell reproduction, the immune system functions poorly, and by retarding the body's natural urge to rid itself of foreign molecules, the doctors give the transplanted organ a chance to take root and begin serving the body in place of the original, defective organ.

Unfortunately, a half-effective immune system opens the body to a wide variety of infections—particularly latent ones, in which the germs or viral particles have been present in the system all along, but have hitherto been kept at bay. Not very surprisingly, herpesvirus is one of the most common latent infections to develop during immunosuppression. Researchers have noted that owing to the reduced immunity in bone-marrow transplant candidates, latent herpesvirus begins to infect the entire system. (In these immuno-compromised patients, the anti-viral drug acyclovir is used effectively against herpesvirus. Acyclovir, now on the market, is being rigorously tested and—as discussed in Chapter 11—does offer some real hope to the treatment of herpesvirus.) In addition, patients being immunosuppressed often develop cancer. In other patients, existing tumors rapidly grow and spread. In these instances, doctors halt the immunosuppression; and if the body is still able to recover, complete remission of the cancer often follows, as the immune system begins doing its job again.

In other words, the immune system *by itself* is an efficient destroyer of cancer cells. If the surveillance is working efficiently, cancers rarely take hold. Only when the immune system functions improperly and too many cancer cells go unattended, or when carcinogenic influences overwhelm the immune system, does this "cellular rebellion" get out of hand. Accordingly, medical science has begun exploring the exciting idea of *immunotherapy*—simply stimulating the immune system to greater efficiency in seeking out and destroying mutant cells. (By contrast, the more traditional cancer treatments of chemotherapy and radiation often kill healthy cells as well as cancerous ones.)

Even in normal patients, the efficiency of the immune system varies greatly from person to person. Recurrence-free individuals may be blessed with more effective immune systems than average. Or a recurrence-free person's immune system may simply have a particularly strong resistence to herpesvirus, while being "normally" weak against the common cold, for example.

As with any other form of physical or mental illness, rate of recovery is very much up to the individual. Mrs. Sloan believes in the concept of wellness and self-responsibility. "Is it your responsibility to be sick or well?" she asked her audience. "How much time do you spend thinking about herpes? If you don't want the disease around, don't be nice to it. Don't be a good host, one of those people who are always saying, 'No, that's okay, you go first; I was just waiting.' Nice people let everything happen to them. Don't be nice to everything; be more selective. Let the disease *know* how you feel. Talk to it: 'I don't want you here. And when you are here, stay for only a little while. Then go, move on, leave me alone.' "

Donald Ardell, Ph.D., editor of the *American Journal of Health Planning*, has written a book *High Level Wellness: An Alternative to Doctors, Drugs and Disease*, which explores such vital dimensions of well-being as nutritional awareness, stress management, fitness, and self-responsibility. Its "Wellness Resource Guide" includes detailed reviews of some 70 other books that will contribute essential knowledge to anyone wanting to enter a state of "high level health." No book we've come across provides a broader and more readable introduction to the concept of being *responsible* for one's own well-being.

We enthusiastically recommend *High Level Wellness* to all herpesvirus patients, because in any case, keeping your resistance as high as possible maintains a second line of defense against herpesvirus—ensuring that whatever recurrences you *do* experience are mild and of short duration. For example, are you certain you're eating a fully-balanced diet that includes all essential vitamins and nutrients? If your body is being deprived of any of the ingredients it needs to maintain optimum health, your immune system is robbed of its ability to function efficiently—and you are much more likely to experience recurrences.

16

Nutrition—Your Personal Route to Higher Immunity

The goal of life is living in agreement with nature. — ZENO

Daniel K.: *Another way I have grown personally through the herpes experience is that I used to be a nutritional illiterate. I knew more about caring for my car than caring for my body.*

Debbie: *This man I liked was into health foods, and he kept going on and on about what he thought might be good for my recurrences. Then we parted company, and the next Monday, nine o'clock sharp, he called, sounding excited. "Do you have a piece of paper?" he asked. "Write this down." He said that he'd been doing a lot of reading over the weekend and that he had a list of vitamins and minerals that he was sure would at least help.*

I felt kind of good because he was taking a helpful interest. He used to nag me—did I get any vitamins yet? Had I tried any herb teas?— maybe just to protect himself. It was a little annoying, but I couldn't be mad at him; I thought it was a hell of a nice way for him to respond. He felt all disease could be controlled through nutrition, and he might be right.

In the past, people had to rely on whatever foodstuffs were available in a given season, and in a particular place. And before the invention of refrigeration and high-speed transportation, only a small variety of food and drink was available in any one part of the country. Today's supermarket carries a greater variety of high-quality, nutritionally varied foods than were available to the wealthiest rulers of 16th century Europe.

Yet in the face of this fabulous edible wealth, many Americans suffer from what the book *Mega-Nutrition* refers to as "chronic subclinical malnutrition." The author, Richard A. Kunin, M.D., dismisses the assertion that the normal American diet is adequately nutritious: "Nothing could be further from the truth," he writes, adding that "the claim that an arbitrary mix of various food types can adequately support the health of widely varying individuals is demonstrably false . . . The assurances we hear from the medical establishment that we can obtain all the nutrients we need from supermarket food are incessant, but unsupported by the facts."

When any bodily system is deficient in any of its components, then clearly it can't function at full efficiency. And some individuals' immune systems do not function optimally because of poor nutrition. "I eat a balanced diet," insist many herpesvirus patients. But do they? According to pharmacist Earl Mindell's classic *Vitamin Bible* (which, by the way, is *not* a religious tract), we humans have to concern ourselves with six important classes of nutrients: carbohydrates, proteins, fats, minerals, vitamins, and water. The *macro*nutrients (carbohydrates, fats, and proteins) supply energy to the body—but only when the proper balance of *micro*nutrients (minerals and vitamins) are present.

What *are* vitamins, exactly? Mindell defines them as, "quite simply, organic substances necessary for life. Vitamins are essential to the normal functioning of our bodies and, save for a few exceptions, cannot be synthesized or manufactured by our bodies. They are necessary for our growth, vitality, and well-being. In their natural state, they are found in minute quantities in all organic food. We must obtain them from these foods or in dietary supplements."

Some critics insist that vitamin and mineral supplements sold in supermarkets, health food stores and via mail order are useless and represent today's version of the snake-oil cures. This opinion holds that our foods already contain all the essential nutrients we need. The other side, however, contends that the micronutrient content of our daily meals has been dramatically reduced. Drs. W.M. Ringsdorf and Emanuel Cheraskin of the University of Alabama School of Medicine demonstrated that from a typical American dinner consisting of pork chops, potato, and vegetables, at least 50 percent of the original vitamins and minerals have been lost.

Our diet gets assaulted in a number of ways. Most food is grown on burned-out farmsoil, exhausted of its trace chemicals and organic matter by overuse and repeated application of chemicals. Fruits and vegetables are routinely transported hundreds of miles from the place they were grown—effectively diminishing much of the vitamin content (and mineral content, to a lesser degree). Storage in the supermarket further delays the time between harvest and ingestion, destroying more vitamins along the way. Washing and peeling removes more of the nutrient-rich outer layer of food. Defrosting food reduces up to 10 percent of the remaining micronutrients, according to *Mega-Nutrition* author Dr. Richard A.Kunin. Actual food preparation probably destroys the most vitamins and minerals of all. The fresher the better; the less cooking the better. Defrosting may be bad, but overcooking is worse. (Boiling spinach, for example, destroys as much as 75 percent of its vitamins.)

Not only do manufacturers go to great lengths to remove the healthful qualities of our food, but they compound the problem by adding dangerous preservatives and substances, many proven to cause cancer in laboratory animals, to "enhance" flavor and appearance. (A moment's reflection will recall that Adam and Eve were not tempted by the apple because its color had been improved with Red Dye No. 2, or because its surface had been rendered more glossy by an application of wax.) In its report *Nutrition and Health: An Evaluation of Nutritional Surveillance in the United States* (1975), the U.S. Senate Select Committee on Nutrition stated that:

> The threat is not beriberi, pellagra, or scurvy. Rather we face the more subtle, but also more deadly reality of millions of Americans loading their stomachs with food likely to make them obese, to give them high blood pressure, to induce heart disease, diabetes, and cancer—in short, to kill them over the long term.

Technically, nutrition may be defined as the science of supplying the body with all the substances needed to perform the biological functions necessary for health. But in practice, nutrition is an art, if you want to maintain an immune system that not only surveys constantly and aggressively for foreign invaders, but also launches an effective attack as soon as it discovers any herpesvirus particle.

Without a complete array of essential nutrients, your body can't go about its biological business of survival. And nutrition, like the proverbial chain, is only as strong as its weakest link. With grateful acknowledgement to Rodale Press of Emmaus, Pennsylvania (publishers of the unexcelled *Prevention* magazine), we reprint here from Dr. Ardell's book *High Level Wellness* his fifteen principles of nutritional awareness:

1. *Go out of your way for natural, "live" foods.* They are usually harder to obtain than convenience or fast foods, but the extra effort is well worth your trouble. A number of especially beneficial foods do more than their fair share to help your body work well. Some highly recommended ones:
   A) *Soybean sprouts,* which can be grown in your kitchen, have an enzyme called invertase that can help convert an otherwise impoverished diet into carbohydrates directly assimilable into usable energy.
   B) *Fresh whole fruits and raw vegetables* are better than the juices, which lose something in the heating process for canning and bottling. They are best of all when taken from your own pesticide-free garden.
   C) *Yogurt,* easy to make and delicious to eat plain or sweetened with honey and/or fresh fruits, facilitates digestion and increases resistance to infections.

D) *Garlic*, an antiseptic that decreases the amount of harmful bacteria in the stomach and reduces blood pressure for those with hypertension, is delicious (and leaves little mouth odor if mixed with or followed by fresh parsley).

E) *Honey*, the "nectar of the gods," preserves vitamins and contains valuable minerals (copper, iron, calcium, sodium, titanium, and potassium). It also contains all 10 essential amino acids, and is a mild laxative, a gentle sedative, and a natural alternative to sugar.

F) *Apple cider vinegar* is both a healing agent and an antiseptic, though I admit it tastes terrible.

G) *Nutritional yeast* contains all the B vitamins in natural form. Some varieties of brewer's yeast are also over 50 percent protein.

H) *Wheat germ*, usually removed from packaged goods to preserve shelf life, has an abundance of Vitamin E, B vitamins, and important trace minerals.

I) *Watermelon*, familiar to nearly everybody, is an excellent diuretic for eliminating toxins.

J) *Sunflower seeds*, loaded with vitamins, minerals, and trace elements, are rich in fiber and are an excellent source of polyunsaturated oil high in linoleic acid. Easy to digest, they taste wonderful alone or in salads.

K) *Bran* has increasingly been recognized as the single most valuable ingredient in promoting a healthy digestive tract.

2. *Vary your diet.* Choose different types of foods throughout the week (milk and dairy products, meats, fish, leafy vegetables, seeds, root vegetables, and fruits), but examine the arguments on the controversial subject of food combinations. Become your own most trusted expert on what is good for you.

3. *Avoid dangerous foods and food additives.* Known and suspected carcinogenic elements enter food as artificial colors, additives, preservatives, stabilizers, and other processed chemicals. An NBC television documentary, "What Is This Thing Called Food?" provided a summary, noting that 5,500 different chemicals go into the U.S. food chain. Nitrates, a leading factor in cancer of the colon, are found in most bacon, sausage, luncheon meats, and frankfurters; and petroleum derivates such as BHA, BHT, and artificial flavors and colors are standard ingredients in many foods. In addition to the hazard of altering meats, fruits, and vegetables through chemical restructuring, neither our government nor the manufacturers have established the safety of these contaminants. These counterfeit products cannot do you any good, so why take chances?

4. *Boycott refined, processed foods.* Packaged cereals, candies, commercial ice creams, colas, etc. consist mostly of empty calories devoid of vitamins, amino acids, and minerals. You have relatively little control over packaging and distribution methods, but you don't have to buy what you know is deficient in needed food ele-

ments. And refined, processed foods are relatively empty products compared with "unmanufactured" fruits, vegetables, certain meats, fowl, dairy products, seeds and grains. In fact, thanks to various processings, as much as 80 percent of the food value in the 3,500 calories the average American eats each day is lost. Don't let the processors fool you with "enriched" milled grain products because thiamine, riboflavin, niacin, and iron have been put back into the product. These foods are as "enriched" as you are when you receive a $100 tax refund after paying out many thousands during the year. The essential nutrients have been mostly taxed away.

5. *Learn to dislike refined carbohydrates.* Sugar provides calories—period. It is absorbed directly into the bloodstream, requiring an immediate insulin treatment from the pancreas, which upsets the endocrine balance within the body. Refined sugar is highly concentrated, lacking other proteins needed for metabolic function. The body must therefore draw on its own reserves to metabolize the sugar, causing a loss of vitamins B_1, B_2, B_6, niacin, magnesium, cobalt, and other substances. If the sugar is not completely metabolized, a buildup of lactic and pyruvic acid can occur that leads to tissue degeneration.

Empty calories are worse than no food at all, for they take the place of other calories that could provide nutritional fuels for hungry cells. Refined sugar has no fiber, which means it does nothing for digestion and a lot for tooth and gum disease. The average citizen may consume 120 pounds of the stuff annually. The story on white flours is similar: the valuable germ and the outer bran coat of wheat are discarded in milling with consequent loss of vital nutrients and the "gain" of empty starches. You can recognize that soda pop, pastries, synthetic ice creams, potato chips, white-flour spaghetti, white bread, and similar cardboard foods probably don't taste as good as you thought they did, especially when tempting and nutritious alternatives are available (honey/molasses, fresh fruits, whole-grain breads, seeds, and all the rest).

6. *Keep it simple and take your time.* It's not necessary to give up supermarkets, grow everything yourself, and transform your food habits overnight. On the contrary, it's best if you make the basic changes as you gradually feel more strongly about the importance of sound diet. Realistic goals help your evolution toward wellness remain a pleasant activity rather than a grind.

7. *Eliminate coffee, tea, alcohol and other addictive drugs.* Not much needs be said about the destructive aspects of alcoholic drinks (including wine) or hard drugs. But coffee and tea (and cola and chocolate drinks) all contain caffeine, which stimulates the sympathetic nervous system, induces acid secretion in the stomach, leads to heartburn, bleeding ulcers, and related disorders. It can keep you from sleeping, make you nervous, rob your body of thiamine, and scald your throat. There's probably only one good

explanation why so many of us drink coffee: it is a drug to which we have become habituated! A high correlation has been found between coffee consumption and illness in general, and the same correlation holds for tea: both utilize stored body sugars from the liver at an excessive rate, alternately raising and lowering blood sugar levels. It's better to enjoy juices, herbal teas, and other substances that nourish rather than draw from your body.

8. *Concentrate on quality in proteins.* Your need for protein varies with your overall state of health, stress level, diet, and your liver's capacity for synthesizing proteins. Protein foods containing all eight essential amino acids are referred to as first-class proteins. They are found in both animal and vegetable products; however, foods containing the essential acids in varying amounts most prefered by the body (*i.e.,* complete proteins) are meats, dairy products, and seafood. Vary your animal and vegetable sources of protein for best effect. If you want to eat economically and ecologically, you don't have to eat foods with complete protein; you can, instead, mix whole grains, legumes, and other inexpensive foods in combination, to obtain what Frances Moore Lappé calls protein complementarity. As in nearly everything else, you are the one who must assess how much protein you need, given your unique lifestyle and energy demands.

9. *Enjoy fresh fruit and uncooked vegetables every day.* The fresher your food, the more enzymes and nutrients are in it. Naturally, the more organic and less cooked your fruits and vegetables, the better. During the Renaissance, it is said that cooks would pick vegetables and *run* to the kitchen.

10. *Try to get high-fiber roughage every day.* Starches, fats, oils, sugars, refined flours, and other extensively purified carbohydrates convert into fecal matter that remains in the lining of your colon for three or four days. This can lead to nausea, heartburn, excessive gas, bloating and distention, abdominal pain, rectal irritation, and constipation. Worse, it can eventually produce degenerative diseases, particularly coronary heart disease, cancer of the colon or rectum, appendicitis, hemorrhoids, diverticulitis, varicose veins, phlebitis, and obesity. So if you need another reason to shun commercial ice creams, white flours, breakfast cereals, hamburgers, hot dogs, refined pastries and desserts, you have it. The best ways to ensure that you get the 24 or so roughage grams recommended daily are to take a teaspoon of two of bran each day, use whole-grain products, enjoy fresh fruits and raw vegetables, and avoid junk food.

11. *Sometimes age-old wisdoms still hold.* You need, for example, to chew your food slowly and thoroughly (this gives fiber time to absorb liquid), to eat only when hungry, to drink lots of water, to get balanced meals (something from each of the four food groups at each meal), and use nature's herbs for natural vitamins and as alternatives to chemical medicines and synthetic pills. Eliminate booze, get a good night's sleep, exercise regularly, and avoid worrying too much.

12. *Take just a moment for reflection with your food.* This needn't be religious reflection, simply a thoughtful mood in which you link eating to your sense of life's meaning and purpose. You might try eating alone occasionally—find a place that feels good and comforts you, take one course at a time, and be unhurried while you enjoy dining with yourself. Much of what we think of as hunger is a desire for attention, sensual pleasure, relief from anxiety, and gratification. Pay special attention to how each morsel tastes, and how it feels when you swallow. You may find this approach helps you avoid eating foods that do little for your health, gaining weight from overeating, or leaving the table tense and unsatisfied. After a while, eating will become a more integrated part of your life, and less a means of entertainment.

13. *Find a friend with whom to share nutritional adventures and discoveries.* Make time for the joy of cooking, the satisfaction of good eating. If you already have a mate interested in nutritional awareness, wonderful. Eating well is seldom accidental; it is hard enough without having to be distracted by a low-level diner.

14. *Keep eating a pleasure, and never an obsession.* You don't have to count calories (vitamin and mineral content is more important), measure portions, or undergo the folderol of weight-watching grinds to be healthy and fit. Just eat sensibly and get plenty of exercise, rest, and enjoyment in life. Be suspicious of quick-weight-loss schemes (results are always temporary), and avoid any diet plan that destroys your enjoyment of food. Do little things that make good food pleasurable. For example, if you are serving fresh apple-strawberry juice, use your most exquisite wine glasses. Psychologically, it makes the transition easier, and can make the juice seem all the more worth savoring.

15. *Start every day with a full, nutritious breakfast.* While you're at it, enjoy a satisfying lunch and dinner. Skipping meals (except when fasting or systematically undereating) often leads to food distractions throughout the day. Don't leave the table hungry. Be aware that little or no breakfast can cause dangerously low blood-sugar levels, interfering with concentration and stimulating you to a junk-food splurge.

The Case for Vitamin Supplements

Even critics of vitamin supplements agree that illnesses and infections make the body use a greater-than-normal quantity of vitamins and minerals. Furthermore, it's suggested that the stress of modern civilization and the increase of toxins in the air and water make our bodies require even greater amounts of nutrients. Therefore, it makes sense for herpesvirus patients to take at least a daily multiple vitamin/mineral supplement in addition to their regular diet.

Dianne R., a 28-year-old field engineering consultant for a computer manufacturer, lives in Houston. She believes she caught herpesvirus from her steady boyfriend, but hasn't suffered a recurrence in almost two years.

Dianne: *In my first and only infection, the pain was so intense I was bedridden. It hurt so much to urinate that I had to do it in a bathtub full of cool water. That worked well, but now it disgusts me to think of sitting down in a tub to take a bath.*

I've never had another infection. I'm not sure why, but when I went to the Herpes Symposium, I got the impression that I'd better start taking care of myself—real good care. I now go to bed early and get up early. I eat better food, too—not so much junk. And I take vitamins: a multi-, and E and A, the B complex, and some minerals.

Jim M. is a 37-year-old graphic designer living in Long Island. He has had genital herpes for two years, but has not had a recurrence for eighteen months, after designing a mega-vitamin therapy program for himself.

Jim: *I had an initial outbreak that seemed to last forever, but was really only a couple of long weeks. A second outbreak—about a month after the first one cleared up—got me nervous. I thought I might be having these attacks every month or so, and I was really down. I tried reading up on herpes, but there wasn't much literature on it. The few articles I did find all seemed to be taken from the same sources—the questions and answers were the same.*

One article, though, said something about how vitamins can keep you healthier and help you resist the infection better. Now there was a lot of good information about vitamins, and I undertook quite a study. I must have read a library and a half of books and articles until I knew what my vitamin and mineral diet was going to consist of. I bought about thirty bucks worth of vitamins at the health-food store—expecting the purchase to last me about a month. A dollar a day was worth it, if it worked.

The owner of the health-food store asked me what I was up to. I didn't tell him about the herpes, just said that I wanted to improve my health. He didn't say anything, but the look he gave me started me thinking. So I asked our family doctor. He said that all vitamins were a waste of money—that a well-balanced diet would supply me with all the vitamins I'd need. But I knew that most of the vitamins in foods are lost in the store or when the restaurant boils them to death. I ignored my doctor and started taking them religiously.

Now I haven't had a recurrence since I began this program, though as I learn more and more about vitamins—it seems there's something new every day—I have changed some of the dosages. Some minerals I didn't need because of my diet. Others I didn't need because I didn't have any problem requiring that vitamin or mineral. It's not good to take something if you don't need it.

I can't say that the vitamin program has prevented my herpesvirus from recurring, but I can't say it hasn't. But I know one thing: I feel better now than I ever did, and I'm getting near age forty! Of course, studying up on vitamins has made me a lot more aware of nutrition in general, so I guess that's part of it. But down deep, I really believe that the vitamins have given me something I didn't have before. I used to get colds all the time—maybe ten times a year, and some of them were unbelievable. The congestion was so bad I could only breathe through my mouth. Now, since all this herpes and vitamin business, I haven't had a cold. I know that doesn't prove anything, but the facts speak for themselves.

For a representative survey of vitamins, minerals, and their role in nutrition, see Appendix B. But for herpesvirus patients, Vitamin C is worthy of particular discussion here—because it's alleged to have definite antiviral properties.

Scurvy, an ailment characterized by muscle weakness, lethargy, and bleeding beneath the surface of the skin, has been described by writers long before the birth of Christ. Antarctic explorer Captain Robert Scott and his party died of this affliction in 1912. Yet as little as 10 mg. a day of Vitamin C—the amount in one slice of orange—is enough to prevent scurvy.

In recent years, Vitamin C (technically known as ascorbic acid) has been the focus of wild claims and furious controversy. Some assertions—that Vitamin C can cure cancer and forestall heart attacks—*are* outlandish. But more reasonable voices who hail the vitamin as a general stimulator of the immune system are shouted down by skeptics unable or unwilling to believe that a non-toxic substance can do so many things simply and inexpensively.

Jim: *The government recommends you take 45 milligrams. I take forty or fifty times that amount—2½ grams a day. Some people take up to 12 grams a day, but if you take too much, you develop diarrhea—that's when you know. But I never took that much. In Linus Pauling's book* Vitamin C and The Common Cold, *he describes how the body's need for C increases when you get sick. They tested the amount of ascorbic acid excreted in urine to determine how much was being absorbed, waited until the people being tested fell ill, and then tested them again. They found that much less ascorbic acid was being lost. The conclusion was that the body uses more Vitamin C when it needs it.*

In the debate over this micronutrient, the name of Linus Pauling keeps cropping up. Few men have won the Nobel Prize even once; but Dr. Pauling won the Nobel Prize for Chemistry in 1954 and the Nobel Peace Prize in 1962. (Later in 1975, as an anticlimax, he was awarded the National Medal of Science.)

Earlier, in 1968, Dr. Pauling stated that "Orthomolecular medicine is the preservation of good health and the treatment of disease by varying the concentrations in the human body of substances that are normally present in the body and are required for health." In his world-famous book, *Vitamin C and the Common Cold* (more recently updated as *Vitamin C, the Common Cold, and the Flu*), Dr. Pauling recounts how medical science refused to acknowledge Vitamin C's substantial disease-resisting qualities. In March of 1975, he reports that the American Medical Association issued a press release titled, "Vitamin C Will Not Prevent or Cure the Common Cold."

The AMA statement was, apparently, based on the results of a controlled study of Vitamin C using employees of the National Institute of Health as subjects. In Dr. Pauling's interpretation of the statistics, "the amount of illness was 20 percent less for the Vitamin C subjects than for the placebo subjects." Tired of the constant, unfair and subjective criticism of studies that disputed his contentions, Dr. Pauling gathered together his best evidence in order to refute the "bad press" that Vitamin C was getting, and directed his reply to the *Journal of the American Medical Association:*

> . . . I at once prepared a thorough but brief analysis of thirteen controlled trials and submitted it to the editor on 19 March. He returned it to me twice, with suggestions for revisions, which I made. Finally, on 24 September, six months after I had submitted the article to him, he wrote to me that it was not wholly convincing and that he had decided to reject the article and not publish it in the *JAMA*. It was later published in the *Medical Tribune* (Pauling, 1976b).

In the chapter, "The Medical Establishment and Vitamin C," Dr. Pauling describes incident after incident of similar behavior by usually responsible medical authorities.

Does ascorbic acid indeed possess definite antiviral properties? As evidence, Dr. Pauling offers the reduced frequency, duration, and severity of the common cold in those persons who increase their intake of Vitamin C. Of course, *any* substance that is alleged to help ward off viruses in general is of great interest to herpesvirus patients. But in addition, Dr. Pauling has had personal experience in treating his late wife's oral herpesvirus infections with both topical and ingested Vitamin C. When we asked Dr. Pauling about the effects of ascorbic acid on herpesvirus lesions, he wrote back as follows:

> In answer to your letter about Vitamin C and herpes simplex, I may say that my wife, Alva Helen Pauling, reported to me about ten years ago that she controlled herpes simplex infections on and around her lips (which developed after she had been working in the garden in the bright sun) by applying ascorbic acid powder or sodium ascorbate powder directly to the lesions. At these times, she was also taking 3 grams per day or 10 grams per day of ascorbic acid by mouth. She said that the lesions healed up very quickly, within a few hours.
>
> I have also recommended topical application and oral ingestion of ascorbic acid or sodium ascorbate to a number of people who wrote to

me about herpes veneralis. I have had some reports of effectiveness, but do not have detailed information.

Does Vitamin C really inhibit viral particles—or simply boost the immune system's ability to combat herpesvirus? Will ascorbic acid work for you? Whether or not you accept Dr. Pauling's conclusions, his fascinating book *Vitamin C, the Common Cold, and The Flu* will, at least, increase your knowledge of the ways that the body can increase its resistance to disease.

Epilogue

A wise person should consider that health is the greatest of human blessings, and learn how by his own thought to derive benefit from his illnesses.
— Hippocrates, *Regimen in Health*, Book IX

William A. Wisdom, Ph.D. is Chairman of the Department of Philosophy at Temple University. He contracted genital herpesvirus several years ago and has been instrumental in establishing the Philadelphia chapter of HELP.

What effect has herpesvirus had on your life?

Dr. Wisdom: *I really believe that herpes has required me to pay more attention to my body and my well-being, to take care of myself in terms of managing stress. Not by seeking to eliminate stressful situations, but by concentrating on areas of my life that provide satisfaction. Like music; I play the banjo.*

Also, I've thought more about my relationships with other people, both in sexual and non-sexual ways. I became involved with the Philadelphia HELP organization—and I appreciate being able to see people move down to lower levels of emotional anxiety. Informing others and helping them gives me a lot of satisfaction; that's why I went into teaching in the first place. The only negative thing that comes to mind is that I sense some impairment of my libido; of being content with more ordinary things. But I don't know if that's a result of the herpes or of the satisfying long-term relationship that began at about the same time I contracted herpes.

Carrie R.: *I have herpes pretty regularly maybe ten or twenty percent of the time, I'm out of commission sexually. And you know what? I've come to accept it, and almost enjoy it. I've found things to replace the sex that I miss.*

Had it not been for the HELP support groups, I doubt I'd have come out of my shell and realized that the world doesn't begin and end with sex. In our group, there's a couple—a husband and wife—who both have herpes, and they were big enough to share some of their non-sexual loving techniques with the group.

There's a whole new world of non-sexual intimacy that I was forced to discover. "Reality is the mother of invention," and I've invented a lot of non-sexual things to do with lovers—close lovers, though. I haven't tried going to a bar, picking up a guy, and coming back to my apartment to try some long, sensuous embraces without engaging in genital contact. I don't know how a stranger would take to that. But old friends and lovers genuinely enjoy it. I'm sure they're sincere. It adds a new dimension to sex, and to relationships in general.

At the support group, I learned to be open, to express myself; and I've carried that ability into other areas of my life. Right now I drive a cab, but in the fall I'm starting grad school. I really believe that my new-found ability to express myself helped me decide to go to school. I know it helped me get accepted. They weren't so impressed with my undergraduate grades or my GRE score. But in the personal interview, that's where I swayed the Director of Admissions in my favor.

Daniel K.: The effect has been pretty significant, I'd say. And it's the truth when I tell you it's been mostly for the good. Don't get me wrong—if I could start over again, I wouldn't want to get it. But since I did, and I admit I had some trouble adjusting to it at first, it's taught me so much more about life in general than I could have imagined.

I'm almost glad I caught herpes. I realize I'm really lucky, believe me. Some people get herpes pretty severely, and so I imagine it's much more difficult to adjust. But through my therapy—which, by the way, I have kept up—I learned a lot about myself that I'm now convinced would have given me plenty of trouble later in life.

I don't think I'll stay in therapy forever, but I was an arrogant person. I didn't take the time to look around very much. I wore blinders. I had a lot of material things, and everything was fine. I would have just glibly traveled down the road of life, almost arrogantly, feeling immortal. But I now see that that kind of existence is what leads to heart attacks and nervous breakdowns and a life of quiet desperation. Catching herpes has helped me slow down.

Having herpes has made me more aware of—I don't know the right word—well, more of everything. I'm happier and healthier than ever before. Herpes was a great cosmic slap in the face, and I really needed it. Through therapy—and remember, it was herpes that brought me into therapy—I've opened up. It has made me more of a whole person. And I don't know if I would have met my girlfriend if I hadn't become something of a different person.

I don't believe that people's fates are predestined. But I do believe that catching herpes was really the best thing that has happened to me. Again, I wish I didn't have it—but I do, and I see it's changed my life. I can't guess whether I'd have eventually developed all of these keen insights into myself without herpes—but I do know it was the catalyst. That's what I mean when I say I'm almost glad I have it.

Sometimes when I think of herpes as that cosmic slap in the face, I want to stand up and shout, "Thanks, I needed that!"

APPENDIX • A
Local Chapters of the Herpes Resource Center

(People who want to know more about the Herpes Resource Center—and receive information about local HRC chapters—should send a stamped, self-addressed envelope to The Herpes Resource Center, P.O. Box 100, Palo Alto, CA 94302.)

Listed below are cities in which local HRC/HELP chapters have been organized.

ALABAMA
Birmingham
Montgomery

ARIZONA
Phoenix

CALIFORNIA
Inland Empire [Los Angeles suburbs]
Long Beach
Los Angeles
Orange County
Sacramento
San Diego
San Francisco/East Bay
San Francisco/South Bay
Santa Barbara
Whittier

COLORADO
Denver

CONNECTICUT
Greater Hartford

GEORGIA
Atlanta

HAWAII
Honolulu

IDAHO
Boise

ILLINOIS
Chicago

KANSAS
Kansas City

LOUISIANA
New Orleans

MARYLAND
Baltimore

MASSACHUSETTS
Boston

MICHIGAN
Detroit
Flint
TriCity [Saginaw/Midland/Bay City]

MINNESOTA
Twin Cities

MISSOURI
St. Louis
Kansas City

NEW YORK
Buffalo
Long Island
New York

NORTH CAROLINA
Triangle [Raleigh/Durham/Chapel Hill]

OHIO
Cincinnati
Cleveland
Columbus
Toledo

OREGON
Portland

PENNSYLVANIA
Philadelphia
Pittsburgh

TEXAS
Dallas
Houston

WASHINGTON
Olympia
Seattle
Tacoma

WISCONSIN
Milwaukee

APPENDIX • B
A Quick Look at Micronutrients

The following survey of vitamins and minerals, what they accomplish and where they are found, is hardly an exhaustive discussion. For more information, there are many excellent books on the subject, and Mindell's *Vitamin Bible* (New York: Warner Books, 1979) is among the best.

Vitamins fall into two main classifications. *Fat-soluble* vitamins such as A, D, E, and K can be stored in the body. The *water-soluble* vitamins, including C and the entire B complex, are not stored and must be replenished regularly.

Vitamin A was the first vitamin ever to be classified, and so was designated by the first letter of the alphabet. One of the fat-soluble vitamins, it is stored in the liver and so need not be consumed every day. Also known as retinol, Vitamin A helps in all sight-related functions—especially in counteracting night blindness. It can also help the body fight off respiratory infections, shorten the duration of disease, maintain healthy tissue and organs, and promote growth of the bones, teeth, gums, and hair. When applied externally, Vitamin A helps heal acne, skin ulcers, and boils. The best single source is liver, but Vitamin A is also found in dairy products, fish liver oils, orange and yellow fruits, and vegetables.

The RDA (recommended daily allowance) is 4,000 international units for women and 5,000 I.U.s for men. But if large quantities of Vitamin A—100,000 I.U.s or more—are taken daily for long periods, serious toxic effects can occur. (Polar bear liver contains so much Vitamin A that it is considered poisonous.) And birth control pills *decrease* the need for this vitamin. If you are on the Pill and feel you need more Vitamin A, consult your doctor.

Vitamin B$_1$ (Thiamin), a water-soluble vitamin, is not stored by the body and must be ingested daily. The disease known as beriberi is a direct result of Vitamin B$_1$ deficiency and is successfully treated by administering doses of B$_1$. It also helps digestion and aids in the functioning of the cardiovascular and nervous systems, thus improving alertness. Thiamin is also used to curb motion sickness and has been tried, with varying degress of success, in treating outbreaks of shingles (herpes zoster).

The RDA is 1.4 mg for men and 1.0 mg for women. The vitamin is non-toxic; excess amounts are simply excreted in the urine. Good sources include cereals, whole-grain products, and meats. Dried yeast, peanuts, many vegetables, milk, and bran all contain at least some thiamin.

Vitamin B_2 (Riboflavin), an easily-absorbed, water-soluble vitamin, is one of the micronutrients essential in the conversion of macronutrients into energy. The body uses greater amounts of this vitamin during times of stress—and obstetricians sometimes recommend slightly increased doses of Vitamin B_2 during pregnancy and lactation. Earl Mindell reports that "America's most common vitamin deficiency is riboflavin." The RDA is 1.6 mg for men and 1.2 mg for women. The best sources are dairy products, green leafy vegetables, meats, liver, and eggs.

Vitamin B_5 (Calcium pantothenate) is a water-soluble vitamin that helps build cells and maintain many central nervous system functions. It plays an important part in converting fats and sugars into glucose and is vital to the normal operation of the adrenal glands. This vitamin also speeds the healing of wounds and is frequently used to treat post-operative shock.

Of particular interest to herpesvirus patients is the crucial role that Calcium pantothenate plays in the production of antibodies. "Pantothenic acid," writes Mindell, "can help provide a defense against a stress situation that you foresee." The RDA is 10 mg for adults. It can be found in meat, whole-grain products, poultry, brewer's yeast, organic foods and green vegetables.

Vitamin B_6 (Pyridoxine), a water-soluble vitamin, is quickly excreted from the body and so needs to be replenished on a daily basis. This vitamin helps metabolize protein and is therefore especially important to herpesvirus patients, who must keep their tissue-regenerative abilities as high as possible.

B_6 is found in nearly all foods, and especially high concentrations appear in meats, brewer's yeast, bran, organic foods, dairy products and whole grains. Lima beans, bananas, and potatoes are also excellent sources. Dietary deficiency is rare, but patients who are being treated with the drug L-Dopa for Parkinson's disease should not take more than the RDA—which is 2.0 mg for adults—because B_6 has been found to interfere with the treatment.

Vitamin B_{12} (Cobalamin), also water-soluble, is sometimes referred to as the "red vitamin." Essential in forming and maintaining red blood cells, B_{12} increases the body's energy and helps the functions of the nervous system. B_{12} has the most complex structure of any vitamin and can be synthesized only by bacteria and microorganisms (plants and animals—including humans—can't produce it). It is stored in the liver, and deficiencies can take up to five years to become apparent. Metabolized best in conjunction with calcium, it is effective in minute doses and is measured in micrograms, not milligrams.

Many claims are made for "megadoses" of B_{12}, but one of the few diseases known to benefit from large doses is pernicious anemia, which physicians treat with injections of this vitamin. The RDA is 3 mcg for adults and 4 mcg for pregnant women. Good sources include dairy products, eggs, beef, liver, kidney, and pork. A note to vegetarians: according to Earl Mindell, "if you . . . have excluded eggs and dairy products from your diet, then you need B_{12} supplementation."

Vitamin B_{13} (Orotic acid) is not licensed for use in the United States, but is available in Europe. There is no RDA, though this vitamin is known to aid in the metabolization of folic acid and Vitamin B_{12}. Researchers believe—though they haven't confirmed—that B_{13} helps reduce the effects of some liver ailments. Good sources include yogurt and root vegetables.

Vitamin B_{15} (Pangamic acid): though there is no essential requirement for this micronutrient, it is known to behave much like Vitamin E—as an antioxidant, but very little research has been conducted in the United States. This is one of the most controversial vitamins around, and the FDA has been studying the possibility of banning the substance altogether until hard data about its effects can be developed. In his *Vitamin Bible*, Mindell describes his personal study of Russian tests of the substance. According to Soviet scientists, B_{15} can extend the lives of cells, neutralize addiction to alcohol, lower cholesterol levels, protect the body against pollutants, aid in synthesis of protein, relieve angina and asthma symptoms, protect the liver from the ravages of alcohol, ward off hangovers, and—of greater importance to herpesvirus patients if subsequent laboratory tests support the Soviet findings—stimulate the immune response.

Vitamin B_{17} (Laetrile), derived from the pits of apricots, is easily one of the most debated vitamins in the world. B_{17} has been touted as an anti-cancer treatment, mostly on the grounds that laboratory animals deprived of this micronutrient seemed to develop tumors at greater rates than control animals. But *adding* B_{17} to the diet does not necessarily prevent or fight cancer. The FDA rejected licensing this vitamin on the grounds that it may be toxic due to its cyanide content, which suggests that cancer patients should not embark on a self-prescribed B_{17} treatment program.

OTHER MEMBERS OF THE B COMPLEX:

Choline acts as a fat emulsifier, helps the liver detoxify the body, and helps break down fats to prevent the buildup of choloresterol. Deficiency can cause cirrhosis of the liver. Some researchers believe that choline also aids memory because of the unique way it is absorbed by the brain. There is no RDA for this substance, although estimated average intake is about 500 mg daily. The best sources of choline are egg yolks, green leafy vegetables, yeast, and organic foods.

Folic acid aids in the formation of RNA and DNA and is essential for proper cellular division and the production of red blood cells. This vitamin has also been shown to improve lactation, and can increase appetite and protect the digestive tract from parasites. It has been shown to stunt the growth of animals deprived of it.

This vitamin is not stored in the body and must be ingested regularly, which explains its fairly high RDA—400 mcg for adults and adolescents, 600 mcg for women lactating, and 800 mcg for pregnant women. The most common sources of folic acid are egg yolks, asparagus, spinach, and broccoli. Fruits and other vegetables are also good sources.

Inositol has been found to assist the body in nourishing brain cells, helping prevent eczema, and lowering cholesterol levels. There is no RDA, but the average adult ingests about 1 gram per day. Good natural sources include fruits, liver, wheat germ, and brewer's yeast.

Niacin has been found to help ease migraine headaches, high blood pressure, and some digestive tract problems. It plays an essential role in the metabolism of proteins, carbohydrates, and fats and is necessary for the synthesis of sex hormones, cortisone, and insulin. The RDA for adults is between 12 and 18 mg. Like other water-soluble vitamins, it is not stored in the body and should be ingested daily. Meat, eggs, milk, dates, figs, avocadoes and prunes are among the best natural sources.

PABA (para-aminobenzoic acid) has important sun-screening properties and, among other things, is used in many suntan lotions. PABA reduces the pain from burns, promotes natural hair coloration, and is essential in maintaining healthy skin. There is no RDA, but this vitamin has no known toxic effects, either. Doses of PABA commonly found in B-complex supplements range from 30 to 1,000 mg. Good natural sources of this B vitamin include wheat germ, brewer's yeast, whole grains, rice, and liver.

Vitamin C (Ascorbic acid) helps synthesize the connective substances that bind cells and other tissues together. It encourages development of teeth and bones, plays an important role in the metabolism of amino acids, aids in the manufacture of hormones and can increase the immune system's resistance to disease. (See page 131 for a full discussion of this significant micronutrient.)

The RDA is 45 mg.—but Vitamin C is a water-soluble substance that is not stored in the body and must be replaced constantly. The best sources of ascorbic acid are the citrus fruits—grapefruit, lemons, limes and oranges. Other fruits include Vitamin C as well—especially apples, strawberries and cantaloupes—as do most leafy vegetables.

Vitamin D, being fat-soluble, is stored in various body tissues, but mostly in the liver. Deficiency results in poor development of teeth and bones, and in a condition known as rickets. It aids in assimilating Vitamin A, is used to treat conjunctivitis, and helps the body utilize calcium and phosphorus. The RDA is 400 I.U. The only foods that provide significant quantities of Vitamin D are fish and fish liver oils. In the United States, Vitamin-D-fortified milk is the principal source. This vitamin is also absorbed through the skin on sunny days; those living in areas heavy with smog and rain receive less sunshine-generated Vitamin D than those residing in bright, clear climates.

Vitamin E (Tocopheral), a fat-soluble vitamin, can be stored in the blood and in many organs for periods as long as several years. One of this vitamin's primary functions is to protect polyunsaturated fatty acids and other vulnerable substances from destructive oxidation. Vitamin E helps the body absorb and utilize Vitamin A, retards the aging of cells, aids in supplying various organs with oxygen, and prevents blood clots. Applied externally, it aids in the healing of burns and helps prevent the formation of scar tissue.

The RDA for Vitamin E is 12 I.U. for women, 15 I.U. for men. Important natural sources are the oils of such vegetables as corn, cottonseed, soybean, and safflower. Eggs, liver, and whole-grain cereals also supply Vitamin E in significant quantities.

Vitamin F is derived from the unsaturated fatty acids in foods. There is no RDA for this substance, but Vitamin F reduces cholesterol deposits in arteries, helps the body utilize calcium, promotes healthy skin, and aids in weight loss by burning up saturated fats. It is known that diets high in carbohydrates (the average American diet, for example) create a need for this vitamin. According to Mindell, the National Research Council suggests that at least 1 percent of one's total calories should come from unsaturated fatty acids. Found in vegetable oils, nuts, and avocadoes, this vitamin is best taken in conjunction with Vitamin E.

Vitamin H (Biotin), actually yet another member of the B complex, is water-soluble. Important in the metabolism of Vitamin C, protein and fat, biotin also helps prevent hair from turning grey, aids in recovery from eczema and dermatitis, and can ease some forms of muscle pain. The RDA for adults is between 100 and

300 micrograms. Some of the best sources are egg yolks, milk, nuts, fruits, and brewer's yeast. If whole raw eggs comprise a large part of the diet, they can impair the body's absorption of biotin, and supplements are recommended.

Vitamin K (Menadione), a fat-soluble vitamin, is important for coagulation (the clotting of blood) and prevents internal bleeding. Deficiencies have been associated with colitis. Aspirin has been shown to destroy the effectiveness of Vitamin K, and mineral oil increases its absorption. There has been no RDA established for Vitamin K, but amounts in excess of 500 mcg are not recommended. Yogurt, eggs, vegetable oils, and green leaf vegetables are excellent sources.

In recent years, two new vitamins have been isolated, but no RDAs have been set—primarily because so little is known about these substances and how they perform within the body.

Vitamin T, known to aid in blood coagulation, can be found in sesame seeds and egg yolks.

Vitamin U, found in raw cabbage, may have significance in treating and healing digestive tract ulcers.

A MINERALS SURVEY

Of the 103 chemical elements known to man, not all are essential to life— but about ninety have been detected in living organisms. Minerals assist the human body in literally all of its functions. Muscle movements, biochemical reactions, and the body's nervous system all come to a halt under conditions of extreme mineral deficiency. Without calcium and magnesium, bones would break and crumble; without iron, the blood could not transport oxygen.

Following is a brief survey of the more important minerals and what they accomplish:

Calcium aids in development of the bones and teeth, in coagulation, muscle contraction, and nerve impulse transmission. RDA is 800 mg. Dairy products and green, leafy vegetables are the best sources.

Chlorine maintains acid-base balance in body fluids and is a component in digestive acids. There is no RDA; this substance is found in most salts, including table salt.

Chromium regulates the concentration of blood sugar. There is no RDA, but adults excrete about 20 to 50 mcg each day. It is found in meats, whole grains and organic foods. Brewer's yeast is an excellent source.

Cobalt is found in Vitamin B_{12}, which see. There is no RDA; the vitamin associated with it is found in dairy products, meats, and seafood.

Copper, an element in the enzymes that produce amino acids and metabolize iron, is essential in the production of hemoglobin. There is no RDA; seafood, liver, and green vegetables are the best sources.

Fluorine is an important micronutrient in maintaining healthy teeth and plays a part in maintaining a sound skeletal system. There is no RDA; tea and seafoods (eaten complete with small bones) are good sources.

Iodine, an integral part of the hormone produced in the thyroid gland, aids in regulating energy in the body. The RDA is 130 mcg for men and 100 mcg for women. Iodized salt and seafood are the best sources.

Iron, found in hemoglobin, helps transport oxygen from the lungs to the rest of the body's cells. RDA is 10 mg for men and 18 mg for women. Red meat and iron-enriched cereals are the best sources.

Magnesium functions in cellular enzyme reactions and is concentrated mostly in bones; it also plays a role in nerve and muscle activity. RDA is 300 mcg for women, 350 mcg for men. It is found in whole grains, cocoa, nuts, peas, and beans.

Manganese is important for healthy bones, nerve function, and reproductive processes. Though there is no RDA, 3 to 6 mg are considered sufficient to maintain health in adults. Good sources include nuts and whole-grain cereals.

Molybdenum, a common component in enzymes, has a role in iron metabolism. There is no RDA: molybdenum is found in many foods and is so common that there is no evidence of any deficiency.

Nickel is thought to function in liver oxidation. There is no RDA; researchers are not sure of its sources in foods consumed by humans.

Phosphorous, found in all cells, is essential in metabolism and is concentrated primarily in the teeth and bones. RDA is 800 mg. Dairy products, meats, peas, beans and whole grains are excellent sources.

Potassium aids in regulating the acid-base balance, nerve impulse transmission, and muscle motion. Though no RDA has been established, most adults should have about 2.5 grams daily. It can be found in citrus fruits, bananas, carrots, tomatoes, and seafoods.

Selenium, an important component in cell membranes, may have a role in protein synthesis. It may also protect the human system from the toxic effects of heavy metals such as mercury, and is believed to help prevent cancer when taken in conjunction with Vitamin E. There is no RDA; it is found in seafood and meat.

Silicon aids in the development of bones and connective tissues, but may not be essential in human nutrition. Therefore, there is no RDA; little is known about its food sources.

Sodium is found in the fluids that surround cells and works with chlorine and potassium to regulate the acid-base balance and participate in nerve and muscle activities. Salt is the main source, though sodium occurs in most foods, particularly meats and cheeses. Average intake ranges from 2.5 to 7 grams daily.

Tin is important for normal growth and tooth development in rats, and is suspected to have a similar role in humans—but research is far from conclusive.

Vanadium promotes reproductive ability in laboratory animals and, like tin, is suspected to play a similar role in human nutrition. Scientists are not sure what food sources contain vanadium.

Zinc plays an essential role in sexual maturation, normal growth, and the healing of wounds. It is also present in many enzymes. RDA is 15 mg. Oysters are the best single source, but all seafoods are rich in zinc. Red meats, cheeses, and whole grains are also good sources.

APPENDIX • C
Suggested Further Reading

Herpesvirus: Background and Recent Treatments

"Herpes: New VD in Town." *Ms.*, Vol. IX, (December 1980), p. 62.

"Herpes Patients Fight Medicine's Empty Cupboard." *Medical World News*, July 23, 1979, pp. 27–28.

"Herpes: the Misery and the Hope." *Changing Times*, Vol. 35, October, 1981, pp. 41–42.

"Herpes-Inhibiting Drug Deployed." *Science News*, July 18, 1981, p. 37.

"Medical News: Promising New Anti-Herpes Agent Being Tested in Humans." *Journal of the American Medical Association*, Vol. 240, (1978), pp. 2231–2232.

American Social Health Association, *The Helper*. Since its inception in July, 1979, this newsletter has been a reliable source of new information for herpesvirus sufferers.

Anderson, F.D., Ushijima, R.N., and Larson, C.L., "Recurrent Herpes Genitalis Treatment with Microbacterium Bovis (BCG)." *Journal of Obstetrics and Gynecology*, Vol. 43, (1974), pp. 797–805.

Blough, H.A. and Giuntoli, R.L., "Successful Treatment of Human Genital Herpes Infections with 2–Deoxy–d–glucose." *Journal of the American Medical Association*, Vol. 241, (1979), pp. 2798–2801.

Callahan, J., "The Herpes Epidemic." *New Times*, June 12, 1978, pp. 48–52.

Chang, T., "Genital Herpes and Type 1 Herpesvirus Hominus." *Journal of the American Medical Association*, Vol. 238, (1977), p. 155.

Clark, M., "Herpes: V.D. of the '80s." *Newsweek*, Vol. 99, (April 12, 1982), pp. 75–76.

Corey, L. *et al.*, "Ineffectiveness of Topical Ether for the Treatment of Genital Herpesvirus Infection." *The New England Journal of Medicine*, Vol. 299, (1978), pp. 986–991.

Danziger, S., "Ice Packs for Cold Sores." *The Lancet*, Vol. 1, (1978), p. 103.

Gold, E. and Nankervis, G.A., *The Herpes Viruses*. New York: Academic Press, 1973. A technical study of herpesvirus.

Guinan, M.E., "Topical Ether and Herpes Simplex Labialis." *Journal of the American Medical Association*, Vol. 243 (1980), pp. 1059–1061.

Hamilton, Richard, *The Herpes Book*. Los Angeles: J.P. Tarcher, 1980: The first book about herpesvirus, written by a San Francisco doctor. Still useful.

Kagan, J., "Herpes: It Can Be Treated—But Not Cured." *Ms.*, January, 1978, pp. 15–16.

Laskin, D., "The Herpes Syndrome." *New York Times Magazine*, February 21, 1982, p. 94.

Milier, J.B., "Treatment of Active Herpes Virus Infections With Influenza Vaccine." *Annals of Allergy*, Vol. 42, (1979), pp. 295–305.

Myers, M.G., Oxman, M.N., Clark, J.E., *et al.*, "Failure of Neutral-Red Photodynamic Inactivation in Recurrent Herpes Simplex Virus Infections." *New England Journal of Medicine*, Vol. 293, (1975), pp. 945–949.

Nahamias, A.J., "Herpes Simplex Virus Infection: Problems and Prospects as Perceived by a Peripatetic Pediatrician." *The Yale Journal of Biology and Medicine*, Vol. 53, (1980), pp. 47–54.

Nahmias, A.J. and Norrild, B., "Herpes Simplex Viruses 1 and 2—Basic Clinical Aspects." *Dermatology*, Vol. 25, (1979), pp. 1–49.

Nahmias, A.J. and Roizman, B., "Infection with Herpes Simplex Virus 1 and 2." *New England Journal of Medicine*, Vol. 289, (1973), pp. 667–674, 719–724, 781, 789.

Nolen, W.A., "Facts About a Stubborn Virus." *McCall's*, Vol. 108, (November 1980), p. 184.

Rawls, W.E., Gardner, H.L., Flanders, R.W., *et al.*, "Genital Herpes in Two Social Groups." *American Journal of Obstetrics and Gynecology, Vol. 110, (1971)*, pp. 682–689.

Simon, F.D., "Coping with Herpes—the V.D. that Recurs." *Essence*, Vol. 12, (April 1982), p. 57.

Smith, R.J., "Drug Shows Promise Against Herpes." *Science*, Vol. 213, (July 31, 1981), p. 524.

Van Gelder, L., "The Terrible Curse of Herpes." *Rolling Stone*, March 4, 1982, pp. 23–24.

Wickett, William H., Jr., *Herpes: Cause and Control*. New York: Pinnacle Books, 1982. Describes most things that trigger herpesvirus recurrences, including a discussion of foods that he believes may cause new attacks.

Zimmerman, D.R., "Self-Treatment of Cold Sores with Ice." *The Lancet*, Vol. 2, (1978), p. 1260.

Basic Biology

Andrews, Christopher, *The Natural History of Viruses*. New York: Norton, 1967. Goes beyond basic virology and may be too complex for the layman.

Asimov, Isaac, *A Short History of Biology*. Garden City, NY: Natural History Press, 1964. A popular science writer surveys the history of biology, discussing the basic mechanisms of cell function and dysfunction along the way.

Curtis, Helena, *Viruses*. Garden City, NY: Natural History Press, 1965. A good introduction to what viruses are all about.

The Diagram Group, *The Human Body*. New York: Facts on File, 1980. A profusely illustrated book about the anatomy and physiology of the human body.

Edelhart, Mike and Lindenmann, J., *Interferon*. London: Addison–Wesley, 1981. A look at the amazing substance that may hold the key to curing herpesvirus and cancer.

Gray, Henry, *Gray's Anatomy: The Illustrated Running Press Edition of the American Classic*. 1901 Edition. Philadelphia: Running Press, 1974. Paperback edition of the famous anatomical work. Helpful in visualizing the nerves that the herpesvirus travels on.

Stress Relief and Psychology

Ardell, Donald B., *High Level Wellness*. Emmaus, PA: Rodale Press, 1977. A thorough guide to wellness that explores a variety of routes toward obtaining health and happiness.

Bennett, E.A., *What Jung Really Said*. New York: Schocken, 1966. An interesting, if not esoteric, approach toward understanding psychological changes like those seen in herpesvirus patients.

Benson, Herbert, *The Mind/Body Effect*. New York: Simon & Schuster, 1974. A study of how thought, feeling and emotion affect physiological functions.

Benson, H., *The Relaxation Response*. New York: William Morrow, 1975. An exceptionally helpful guide to reducing stress and anxiety.

Burns, David D., *Feeling Good*. New York: Morrow, 1980. The title says it; a fine book.

Carrington, Patricia, *Freedom in Meditation*. Garden City, NY: Anchor Press/Double-day, 1977. A good book that deals not only with meditation techniques, but also discusses the philosophy of a less-anxious lifestyle.

Cousins, Norman, *Anatomy of an Illness as Perceived by the Patient*. New York: W.W. Norton, 1979. A personal account of the relationship between positive attitude and serious disease. Inspiring—an important book for herpesvirus patients.

Flach, Frederic F., *The Secret Strength of Depression*. Philadelphia: Lippincott, 1974. A good popular psychology treatment of how to turn negative energy into positive energy.

Luce, Gay Gaer and Segal, Julius, *Sleep*. New York: Coward-McCann, 1966. Everything the herpesvirus sufferer will want to know about sleep.

McDonald, Paula and McDonald, Dick, *Guilt-Free*. New York: Grosset and Dunlap, 1977. Useful for herpesvirus patients in helping to eliminate guilt feelings often associated with the virus.

Newman, Mildred *et al.*, *How to Be Your Own Best Friend*. New York: Ballantine Books, 1974. A pop psychology book that is helpful in getting us out of the boxes we often in-advertently put ourselves into.

Pellietier, K.R., *Mind as Healer, Mind as Slayer*. New York: Delta, 1977. An excellent treatise on the brain's ability to create and prevent disease.

Selye, H., *The Stress of Life*. New York: J.B. Lippincott, 1974. A general study of the things that create stress. Herpesvirus patients will especially benefit from the sections on self-induced stress.

Selye, Hans, *Stress Without Distress*. New York: Signet, 1974. Dr. Selye is considered the father of the science of stress. This book is a classic.

Wilson, John R., *et al.*, *The Mind*. New York: Time-Life Books, 1964. An introduction into the science of the mind, offering insight into patterns of thought and behavior that could improve herpesvirus patients' emotional health.

Woolfolk, R.L., and Richardson, F.C., *Stress Sanity and Survival*. New York: Simon & Schuster, 1978. An excellent source book about stress.

Nutrition

"Vitamin C and Immune Protection." *Science News*. Vol. 115, (1979), p. 295.

Airola, Paavo, *Are You Confused?* Phoenix: Health Plus, 1971. A noted nutrition expert wades through many theories on diet and draws some interesting conclusions.

Arlin, Marian T., *The Science of Nutrition*. New York: MacMillan, 1972. Technical details of nutrition and health presented in simple language.

Benowicz, Robert J., *Vitamins and You*. New York: Grosset and Dunlap, 1979. A thorough examination of the body's use of and need for vitamins.

Brody, Jane, *Jane Brody's Nutrition Book*. New York: Norton, 1981. A complete nutrition program in non-technical language.

Consumers Guide (eds.), *The Vitamin Book*. New York:

Faelton, Sharon, ed., *The Complete Book of Minerals for Health*. Emmaus, PA: Rodale, 1981. An introduction to micronutrients (other than vitamins) necessary to maintain health.

Howe, Phyllis Sullivan, *Basic Nutrition in Health and Disease*. Philadelphia: Saunders, 1976. Encyclopedic in scope; an excellent reference book for nutrition and health.

Kunin, Richard A., *Mega-Nutrition*. New York: McGraw-Hill, 1980. One of the best books we've seen on health. Improvement is almost guaranteed by learning and ap-plying the principles of nutrition outlined in this book.

Lappe, Frances Moore, *Diet for a Small Planet.* New York, Ballantine Books, 1975. A good book on how to meet nutrition requirements healthfully and economically.

Milman, N., Scheibel, J. and Jesson, O., "Failure of Lysine Treatment in Recurring Herpes Simplex Labialis." *The Lancet,* Vol. 2, (1978), p. 942.

Mindell, Earl, *Vitamin Bible.* New York: Warner Books, 1979. A complete survey of the vitamins and minerals necessary to maintain a high level of immunity to disease.

Pauling, Linus, *Vitamin C and the Common Cold.* San Francisco: W.H. Freeman, 1970. The winner of two Nobel Prizes documents the disease-preventing qualities of common, inexpensive Vitamin C. An important work for every herpesvirus patient.

Pelletier, Kenneth R., *Holistic Medicine.* New York: Delacourte/Lawrence, 1979. This book explains how to treat patients as human beings, not simply collections of symptoms.

Reuben, D., *Everything You Always Wanted to Know About Nutrition.* New York: Simon & Schuster, 1978. The sex author tries his hand at nutrition. Though we disagree with some of Dr. Reuben's conclusions about vitamin supplements, the book is worth reading.

Samuels, Mike and Bennett, H., *The Well-Body Book.* New York: Grosset and Dunlap, 1975. A wonderful guide to good health and fitness.

Wright, Jonathan V., *Dr. Wright's Book of Nutritional Therapy.* Emmaus, PA: Rodale Press, 1979. A good introduction to improving health through heightened nutritional awareness.

Pregnancy

"Screening Newborns." *Child Today,* July/August 1980, p. 32.

Brewer, Gail Sforza, Ed., *Pregnancy-After-30 Workbook.* Emmaus, PA: Rodale, 1978. Dispells many myths about older mothers.

Colman, Arthur D. and Colman, Libby, *Pregnancy: The Psychological Experience.* New York: Herder and Herder, 1972. A good book for pregnant herpesvirus patients worried about the health of their babies.

Hensleigh, P.A., Glover, D.B., and Cannon, M., "Systemic Herpesvirus Hominis in Pregnancy." *The Journal of Reproductive Medicine,* Vol. 22, (1979), pp. 171–176.

Nance, Sherri, *Premature Babies: A Handbook for Parents,* New York: Arbor House, 1982. An excellent book—important reading for pregnant women suffering from herpesvirus.

Whitely, R.J. and Nahmias, A.J., *et al.,* "The Natural History of Herpes Simplex Virus Infection of Mother and Newborn." *Pediatrics.* Vol. 66, (1980), 489–494a.

Cancer

Hollinshead, A.C. and Knaus, W.A., "Herpes Viruses—A Link in the Cancer Chain?" *Chemistry,* Vol. 50, (1977), pp. 17–21.

Kintzing, J.M., "Too Much Sex Too Soon and Cervical Cancer." *Mademoiselle,* Vol. 86, (April 1980), p. 93.

Prescott, D.M., *Cancer: the Misguided Cell.* New York: Pegasus, 1973. Presents the causes of cancer and the prospects for controlling it.

Glossary

allergy An exaggerated reaction to substances that have no comparable effect on the average individual.

antibodies Proteins created by the immune system that combine with specific antigens and neutralize toxins.

antigen Any substance foreign to the body that stimulates production of antibodies.

antioxidant A substance that prevents or delays deterioration caused by oxygen.

anti-viral drugs Drugs designed to inhibit or destroy virus particles or cells invaded by virus particles.

active immunity Immunity occuring because of prior exposure to infection.

acyclovir An anti-viral drug designed to inhibit replication of herpes simplex viruses. It is the first herpes drug licensed in the United States for use in genital herpes. Acyclovir's effectiveness is the subject of ongoing research.

apthous stomatitis See **canker sores**

argenine An amino acid that has, in the laboratory, promoted the growth of herpesvirus particles.

ascorbic acid Chemical name for Vitamin C.

asymptomatic Being infectious without having symptoms of disease.

autoimmunity An error of the immune system in which an organism develops antibodies against its own cells or tissue; can result in allergy or more serious disease.

autoinoculation The spread of infection from one part of the body to another.

axon A usually long, single nerve cell that transmits nerve impulses.

B-lymphocytes (B-cells) Defensive white blood cells that circulate in the blood and lymph systems and "wait" in lymph nodes in case of antigen attack. Upon discovering an antigen, some B-lymphocytes are transformed into plasma cells.

bacteriophages Cells that consume bacteria.

BCG Bacillus Calmette-Guerin vaccine, which produces antibodies against tuberculosis but is ineffective against herpesvirus.

benign Said of a tumor: not malignant, not recurrent; being favorable for recovery.

biopsy The removal and examination of tissues, cells, or fluids from living organisms.

birth canal The vagina; the path the neonate travels from the womb to the outside world.

blister See **vesicle**.

bone marrow A vascular tissue that fills the cavities of bones.

boric acid An antiseptic salt often used in solution form as a drying agent.

Bowen's disease Cancer of the penis, which may possibly be caused by dye-light therapy, which was once used to treat genital herpesvirus.

Burrow's solution   A solution used topically as a drying agent.

canker sores   Small painful mouth ulcers; apthous stomatitis. Not caused by herpesvirus but often mistaken for oral herpes infection.

capsid   A shell of protein that protects a virus's nucleic acid.

carcinogenic   Cancer-causing.

cauterize   To destroy tissue by burning.

CDC   The Centers for Disease Control, a federal health organization in Atlanta, GA.

cell-mediated immunity   Acquired immunity in which lymphocytes predominate.

cellular immunity (cellular theory of immunity)   The theory of acquired immunity in which thymus-originated white blood cells are the predominant component. See **humoral immunity.**

cervix   The neck of the uterus, located in the upper part of the vagina.

chickenpox   A childhood disease caused by varicella-zoster virus, one of the five members of the herpes family.

chromosome   A structure found in the cell nucleus which "programs" the growth and development of new cells.

clitoris   A small, elongated erectile body in the female; homologous with the male penis.

cold sore   A herpesvirus infection usually occuring on the lip or mouth. Also known as **fever blister, sun blister, herpes labialis.**

colposcope   A binocular-shaped device for examining the cervix and vagina.

conjunctivitis   An inflammation of the mucous membrane lining the inner surface of the eyelids and the front of the eye.

controlled study   See **placebo-controlled double-blind study.**

cornea   The transparant part of the coat of the eyeball that covers the iris and pupil and admits light into the eye.

cortisone   A hormone secreted by the adrenal glands.

culture   (**cell culturing, taking a culture**) The propagation of microorganisms or living tissue cells in a medium that encourages growth.

cryosurgery   Destruction of tissue by application of extreme cold.

cytomegalovirus (CMV)   The least-known member of the five herpesviruses—extremely rare, but generally fatal in infant and neonates.

cytopathologist   A scientist who studies cells and structural changes in cells.

dermis   The inner layer of the skin, below the epidermis.

DMSO   Dimethyl sulfoxide—a skin penetrating solvent.

DNA   Deoxyribonucleic acid—a complex nucleic acid that contains genetic information.

dormant   Latent, or in suspended animation; in effect, asleep.

double-blind study   See **placebo-controlled double-blind study.**

drying agent   A chemical solution applied topically to promote healing by drying the area, reducing the possibility of secondary infection.

dye-light therapy   See **photoinactivation.**

encephalitis   Literally, inflammation of the brain.

enzymes   Complex substances produced by living cells to facilitate bodily biochemical reactions.

epidermis   The outermost, external layer of the skin; the body's largest organ.

Epstein-Barr Virus (EBV)   One of the five members of the herpes family. It causes infectious mononucleosis, also known as "mono" or "kissing disease."

extinction   In Rogerian psychology, the elimination of a behavior.

FDA   The Food and Drug Administration, a federal agency.

fever blister   Herpes labialis, cold sore, sun blister.

ganglion   A mass of nerve tissue containing nerve cells external to the brain or spinal cord.

gene   An element of germ plasm that transmits hereditary information.

genetics   The branch of biology dealing with an organism's hereditary.

genital   Of, related to, or being a sexual organ.

gonorrhea   A sexually transmissible disease—second in incidence only to herpes in the United States.

hepatitis   A disease marked by extreme inflammation of the liver.

herpes progenitalis   Herpes simplex virus I or II infections of the genitals.

herpes simplex I (HSV I)   and

herpes simplex II (HSV II)   Two of the five members of the herpesvirus family. Both viruses cause labial and genital herpesvirus infections.

herpes zoster   Also known as varicella-zoster virus, it causes chickenpox in children and shingles in adults. When varicella-zoster occurs in adults, it is characterized by painful sores on the skin at nerve endings. Shingles, like other herpesviruses, can recur.

herpesvirus   A family of five viruses: **herpes simplex I, herpes simplex II, varicella-zoster, Epstein-Barr** and **cytomegalovirus:** which see.

hormones   Products of living cells that circulate in the body, affecting other cells in other parts of the body.

host   Any organism invaded by a parasite. For example, a skin cell when invaded by a herpes simplex virion.

humoral immunity (humoral theory of immunity)   The theory of immunity in which circulating antibodies—acquired through previous contact with antigens—predominate. See **cellular immunity.**

hypersensitivity   An abnormal or excessive sensitivity; an exaggerated immune response to a foreign substance.

hysterectomy   Surgical removal of the uterus.

IF   *See* **interferon.**

immune   Not susceptible; having or producing antibodies to a given antigen.

immune response   The collective effort of the body to fight disease.

immune system   The body's organization of physiological and biochemical activities that work together to protect the body from foreign substances.

immunity   The condition of being able to resist a particular disease.

immunize   To make an organism immune to a specific antigen.

immunocompromised   The weakening of an organism's immune system by some force such as chemotherapy.

immunodeficient   An immune system that is weak and therefore fights infections inefficiently.

immunopotentiators   A group of drugs used to stimulate immune response beyond normal levels of reaction.

immunosuppression   The process of weakening an organism's immune system for a specific reason, such as preparing a patient for an organ transplant. A normal immune system would reject the transplanted organ as foreign.

immunotherapy   Any treatment to bolster a weakened immune system, or to stimulate a normal immune system beyond its natural limits.

impotence   The state of being unable to achieve penile erection.

infection   In virus diseases, the invasion and establishment of an antigen in a host.

inflammation   A protective tissue response to injury or infection that destroys and walls off both the infection and the damaged tissue.

interferon   An anti-viral substance secreted by cells to prevent viral invaders from attacking neighboring cells.

interferon inducers   Substances that stimulate cells to make and secrete interferon.

initial outbreak   The first herpes simplex virus infection in an organism. Initial outbreaks are usually the most severe because the immune system has not previously "experienced" herpes simplex virus and may take up to ten days to develop antibodies against it.

iris The colored portion of the eye surrounding the pupil.

keratitis Inflammation of the cornea. Often, but not always, caused by herpesvirus.

kissing disease See **Epstein-Barr Virus.**

labia Lips, usually referring to the lips of the vagina—except in herpes labialis which refers to the lips of the mouth.

latency Herpesvirus particles are latent while they are in the ganglia or neural pathways. They are active when they migrate to the skin's surface and invade cells in order to reproduce. See also **dormant.**

lesion A sore or ulceration. Lesions result when herpsevirus particles attack many cells in a single area.

lumbo-sacral ganglion A nerve root at the base of the spine where virus particles from genital herpes infections reside.

lymph gland, lymph node A rounded mass of lymphoid tissue that produces and stores defensive cells that circulate in the lymph and blood systems.

lymphocytes White blood cells which attack and destroy antigens; fundamental to the operation of the immune system.

lymphoma A tumor of lymphoid tissue.

lysine An amino acid whose presence may retard herpesvirus growth.

lysis The process of cell disintegration.

macronutrients Nutrients the body requires in relatively large amounts: fats, proteins and carbohydrates, for example.

macrophages ("great cell eaters") An important component of the immune system, these defensive white blood cells mature in bone marrow and digest antigens and cells invaded by antigens when released into the bloodstream.

malignant Said of tumors: tending to become progressively worse; tending toward death.

micronutrients Organic compounds (like vitamins and minerals) that the body needs in small amounts.

"mono" See **Epstein-Barr Virus.**

mucous membrane A membrane that lines body passages and cavities that communicate directly or indirectly with the exterior.

mucus A viscid, slippery secretion that moistens and protects mucous membrane.

neonate A newborn.

neoplasm A new tissue growth that serves no physiologic function.

nerve pathways See **neural pathways**

neural pathways The routes taken by nerve impulses to or from the ganglia, and, ultimately to the brain.

neuralgia The radiation of pain along nerves.

neurology The scientific study of the nervous system.

neuron A specialized nerve cell.

non-specific immune stimulator A substance that stimulates the entire immune system, not just against a specific antigen.

nucleic acid An acid composed of a sugar or sugar derivative, phosphoric acid and a base. Usually found in cell nuclei.

nucleus The control center of a cell. It contains chromosomes and other genetic data.

outbreak See **initial outbreak** and **recurrence.**

Pap smear A method of examining cervical cells to determine the presence of cancerous or pre-cancerous conditions.

parasite An organism that lives upon or within another organism at whose expense it obtains some advantage.

passive immunity Immunity acquired through the transfer of antibodies.

phagocytes Any defensive cells that ingest disease-causing micro-organisms.

photoinactivation therapy An ineffective and dangerous attempt to treat genital herpesvirus infections.

pituitary gland A small oval endocrine organ attached to the brain that produces various internal secretions necessary for most basic bodily processes.

placebo A pharmaceutically inactive substance—sometimes a sugar pill—given to satisfy a patient's psychological need for treatment. Also used in controlled studies to test the efficacy of medicines.

placebo-controlled double-blind study Usually a study to determine the effectiveness of a new drug, in which neither researchers nor subjects know who is receiving the drug and who the placebo.

plague An epidemic disease causing a high rate of mortality.

primary attack See **initial outbreak.**

prodrome Feelings or sensations that occur before a disease's onset.

rabies An acute viral infection of the nervous system. One of the few virus diseases that can be transmitted from one species to another.

receptor A cell or a part of a cell that has a specific affinity for a particular antibody or virus.

recombinant genes Genes that have been intentionally altered to create new, inheritable characteristics.

recurrences An infection of herpesvirus subsequent to the initial out-break—caused by the migration of herpes virions from nerve ganglia to the skin's surface.

reinforcement In Rogerian psychology, encouragement and incentive to continue a desirable behavior.

replication The process of viruses reproducing themselves.

reportable disease A disease which, by law, must be reported to health authorities whenever a doctor diagnoses it. Syphilis, hepatitis, and gonorrhea are examples of reportable diseases; herpesvirus is not.

RNA (ribonucleic acid) A complex nucleic acid similar to DNA that acts as a transmitter of information in the genetic processes.

saline solution A salt solution used to temporarily maintain living tissues or cells.

Schwann cells Cells that some researchers believe are used by herpesvirus particles as a means of travel to and from nerve ganglia.

scrotum The skin sack enveloping the testicles.

secondary infection An infection by a pathogen following an infection by another pathogen.

shaping In Rogerian psychology, the modification of behavior toward a desired result.

shedding See **viral shedding.**

shingles See **herpes zoster.**

smallpox An acute infectious disease marked by sustained high fever and sores resulting in small, depressed scars.

Sodium ascorbate An acid-free form of Vitamin C.

STD Sexually transmissable disease.

stress Any stimulus that causes the body to react. It may originate internally or externally.

subclinical A condition or disease that exists but is not observable by usual tests or examinations.

subdermal Below the dermis layer of the skin.

steroids Complex compounds (like hormones and cortisone) that are sometimes used topically to treat genital herpesvirus infections, but may only cause the virus to spread.

syphilis A sexually transmissible disease caused by a spirochete. It's treatable with antibiotics, but fatal if ignored.

T-lymphocytes (T-cells) Cells that mature in a tiny neck gland (the thymus) and rush to the site of infections signalled by the biochemical reactions of the immune system. T-cells poison antigens, and attract and motivate macrophages to join the battle against the foreign invaders.

GLOSSARY

tissue   An aggregate of cells that form a structure in plants and animals.

topical   Designed for local application on the surface of the skin or mucous membrane.

trigeminal ganglion   A nerve root in both sides of the face near the temples, where dormant labial and facial herpesvirus particles reside.

trigger   A phenomenon such as stress, sunlight, wind, moisture, friction, trauma that precipitates a herpesvirus recurrence.

tumor   An abnormal mass of tissue that has no physiologic function.

ulcer   A small "crater" on the skin formed as a result of a blister, sore, or infection.

ultraviolet rays   Light rays emitted by the sun that may cause recurrences of labial or facial herpesvirus infections in some people.

urethra   The tube through which urine flows out of the body. It is in the front of the vagina in women and in the penis in men. In men, semen is ejaculated through the urethra.

uterine cervix   See **cervix.**

vaccination   The method of causing the body's immune system to develop antibodies to a specific antigen—usually without introducing a dangerous bacteria or virus into the body.

vaccine   The substance used in vaccination. See **vaccination.**

Varicella-zoster virus (VZV)   See **herpes zoster.**

vesicle   A small blister filled with liquid. Herpesvirus vesicles are extremely contagious.

vesicular fluid   The fluid that collects in a blister.

viral shedding   The activity during (or right before and just after) a herpesvirus infection in which microscopic virus particles are present on the surface of the skin.

viricide   A substance used to kill or retard development of viruses.

virions   Virus particles in their inert, dormant state. Until entering a "host" cell, virions are latent or dormant.

virologist   A scientist who studies viruses.

virus   The Greek word for poison. For our purposes, a virus is a particle that invades cells and causes disease.

Whitlow   Herpetic Whitlow is the name of the infection doctors, dentists and dental hygienists often get on their fingers as a result of contracting herpesvirus—usually from a patient.

white blood cell   A colorless blood corpuscle whose chief function is protecting the body from disease-causing microorganisms; also called a leukocyte. White blood cells originate in bone marrow as undifferentiated cells and take on specific immune functions depending upon where they mature. They can develop into macrophages, B-lymphocytes, T-lymphocytes, or plasma cells.

Zovirax®   Brand name for acyclovir.

Index

chromium, 142
cobalt, 142
copper, 142
fluorine, 142
iodine, 142
iron, 142
magnesium, 142
manganese, 143
molybdenum, 143
nickel, 143
phosphorous, 143
potassium, 143
selenium, 143
silicon, 143
sodium, 143
tin, 143
vanadium, 143
zinc, 143
Moisture, herpes simplex virus and, 15
Molybdenum, 143
Mononucleosis, 22-23, 68, 87
Mount Sinai Hospital, 81
Mucous membranes, herpes simplex virus and, 24, 75
Mumps, 21, 118
Muscle aches, 22, 28
    weakness, 64
Mutations, artificial, 89
Mycalog, 81

Nahmias, Dr. Andre, 16
National Genital Herpes Symposium, 35
National Institue of Allergy and Infectious Disease, 93
National Institute of Health, 89, 93, 132
Natural selection, 31
Neonates, 14, 17, 23, 73-76, 86
    drugs for, 86
    herpes simplex virus and, 17, 23, 28, 72-76
    isolation of, 76
    kissing of, 76
Neoplasms, 66
Nervous system, 14, 22-23, 30-31, 64
    axons, 30, 32
    peripheral cells, 30
    damage to, 17, 72
    ganglia, 22, 30, 37, 62, 64
    pathways, 22
    roots, 30
Neural pathways, 30
Neuralgia, 99
New England Journal of Medicine, 88
New York Magazine, 112
New York University, 47
New Yorker, The, 83
Newborns, *see* neonates
Niacin, 140
Nickel, 143
Nitrates, 126
Nucleic acids, 19
Nuns, cancer and, 67
Nutrition, 122-133, 146
    empty calories, 126
    principles of, 125
    suggested readings in, 146
*Nutrition and Health: An Evaluation of Nutritional
    Surveillance in the U.S.*, 125

Ocular herpes, 14, 17
Oedipus Rex, 35
Ointments, 103
Olson, Kiki, 51
On Becoming a Person, 44
Organ transplants, immunity and, 119
Orotic acid, 139
Orthomolecular medicine, definition of, 131
Outbreak: A Recurrent Newsletter, 50

PAA, 90
PABA, 140
Pain, 22, 98, 102-104
Pangamic acid, 139

Pantothenic acid, 139
Pap smear, 17, 57, 69-71
Papanicolaou, Dr. George, 69, 71
Para-aminobenzoic acid, 140
Paranoia, 42
Parkinson's disease, Vitamin B₆ and, 139
Pasteur, Louis, 117
Pauling, Linus, 131-133
Pauling, Alva Helen, 132
Penis, 13, 82
    cancer of the, 80
Pennsylvania, University of, 62, 91
Pennsylvania State University College of Medicine, 80
Perineum, 104
Peptic ulcers, stress and, 108
Personality changes, 42, 64
Phagocytes, 27-28
Phosphonacetic acid, 90
Phosphorous, 143
Photophobia, 63
Pinkeye, 63
"Pins and needles," feeling of, 99
Pituitary gland, 107
Placebos, 82-84
    studies using, 83
Placenta, 72
Plasma cells, 29
Pneumonia, viral, 21
Polio, 21, 94, 118
Potassium, 143
"Power of the Empty Pill," 84
Pox, 116
Pregnancy, 17, 23, 41, 70, 147
    herpes simplex virus and, 17, 38, 72-76
    premature delivery and, 74
    suggested readings in, 147
Preservatives, cancer and, 125
Prevention, herpes simplex virus and, 51, 94-101
Primates, cancer in, 67
    testing of IC:LC on, 89
Prodrome, 25, 59, 75, 98-100, 114, 116
    symptoms of, 98-99
    treatment for, 104
Produce, fresh, 125
Prophylactics, 97
Prostitutes,
    cancer and, 67
    herpes simplex virus and, 95-96
Protein, 19, 124, 128
    molecules, 19
    quality of, 128
Psychoanalysis, 43
"Psychological Responses to Genital Herpes," 35
Psychosexual development, 35
Psychosomatic disease, 108
Psychotherapy, 43-50
Psychopathology, 42
Pyridoxine, 139
Rabbits, herpes simplex virus and, 20, 30, 79
Rabies, 20, 118
Rapid Eye Movement (REM), 112
Rapp, Dr. Fred, 35, 80, 92
Rash, 22
RDA, 138
Receptors, 21, 24
Recombinant DNA, 89
Recommended Daily Allowances, 138-143
Recurrences, 16, 17, 22, 30, 36-39, 56, 58, 94, 102,
    113-114
    easing discomfort and frequency of, 102-110
    placebos and, 82-84
    pregnancy and, 75
    prevention through hypnosis of, 113-114
    sites of, 24, 31
    trauma-induced, 106
    triggers of, 15, 105-108
    vitamins and, 130-131
Referrals, psychiatric, 41
Relapse, definition of, 23

Relationships, avoidance of, 41, 46
Relaxation, physical effects of, 113-114
Replication, viral, 24, 28, 31, 80
    antiviral drugs and, 84-85
Respiratory tract, 21
Rheumatic fever, 119
Ribavirin, 84
Riboflavin, 139
Ribonucleic acid, 19-20, 24, 67, 84,
    drugs and, 84
Rich, Marvin, 67
Richardson, Frank G., 108
Ringsdorf, Dr. W.M., 124
RNA, *see* ribonucleic acid
Rogers, Carl, 44
Rolling Stone, 51
Rosch, Dr. Paul J., 108
Rouche, Berton, 83
Roughage, 128
Rous, Dr. Francis P., 20, 67
Rous Sarcoma Virus, 20
Russell, Christine, 100

Sabin, Dr. Albert, 80
Sanity and Survival, 108
Scabs, formation of, 13, 29
Scarring, herpes simplex virus blister, 104
Science Digest, 84
Scheie Eye Institute, 62, 91
Scott, Captain Robert, 131
Schwann cells, 30
Scurvy, 131
Seasons, herpes simplex virus and, 106
Selenium, 143
Self-help centers, 35
Self-image, herpes simplex virus and, 37
Self-responsibility, well-being and, 120
Self-treatment, dangerous, 81
Seliger, Susan, 112
Selye, Dr. Hans, 106-107
Sex, 15, 16, 67, 69, 106
    cancer, relationship to, 67, 69
    inability to have, 16
    informing others about herpes before having, 59
    libido and, 134
    postponing of, while infectious, 39, 51-52, 58,
        95, 134
    recurrences and, 37-39, 95-96, 106, 109
Shaffer, Martin, 114
Shakespeare, William, 112
Shapiro, Dr. Arthur K., 83
Shedding of virus particles, 14, 63, 75, 98
Shingles, 21-22, 84, 87
Shipman, Dr. Charles, 86
Silcadene, 81
Silicon, 143
Simian virus, 67
Sitz baths, 103
Sleep, effect of stress on, 42, 112
Sloan, Eleanor C., 36, 40, 43, 121
Smallpox, 21, 81, 116-117
Sobel, Dr. David, 84
Society for Pediatric Research, 100
Socrates, 111
Sodium 143
Sodium ascorbate powder, 132
Sophocles, 35
Sore throat, 22
Soybean sprouts, 125
Spermicides, 81
Spinal cord, 30
Spinal meningitis, 64-65
Spleen, enlarged, 23-24
Stomach, acid secretion in, 127
Stoxil, 63
Steroid creams, 81
Strep throat, 22
Streptococcus, 119

Stress,
    behavior, learned and, 112
    cholesterol and, 108
    effects of sleep on, 40, 112
    General Adaptation Syndrome, 106, 111
    hormones and, 107
    hydrochloric acid and, 108
    peptic ulcers and, 108
    physiology of, 106-107
    psychology of, 15, 111-115
    readings about, 145
"Stress Can Be Good For You," 112
Stressor, definition of, 111
Strokes, 108
Suicide, thoughts of, 16, 42, 44
Sunflower seeds, nutrition in, 126
Sunlight, herpes simplex virus and, 15, 106
Supermarkets, 123-125
Surgery, laser, 80
SV-40, 67
Syndrome, definition of, 98
Syphilis, 47, 51, 67, 96, 116

T-cells, 27-28, 91, 118
T-lymphocytes, 26-28, 91, 118
Tampons, 104
Tea, 127-128
Tetanus, 118
Thiamin, 138
Thoreau, Henry David, 86
Thymidine kinase, 86
Time Magazine, 86, 89
Tin, 143
Tingling, 25, 99
Tocopherols, 141
Topical treatments, 79-81, 103, 132
Toxicity, of antiviral drugs, 90
Trans-placental infection, 73
Transmissability, 23, 28, 100
Trauma, recurrences and, 106
Treatments, 79-93
Trichomonas, 70
Trigeminal ganglion, 30, 62, 64
Truppin, Dr. Michael, 80
Tuberculosis, 81
Tumors, 66
Twain, Mark, 94
2-deoxy-D-glucose (2-DG), 91
Typhoid, 118

Ultraviolet radiation, 106
U.S. Department of Health and Human Services, 79
U.S. Senate Select Committee on Nutrition, 125
Universities:
    Emory University, 16
    New York University, 47
    Pennsylvania State University College of
        Medicine, 80
    Temple University, 134
    University of Alabama, 81, 124
    University of Bologna, 114
    University of California,
        at Los Angeles, 82, 100
        at San Francisco, 24
    University of Michigan, 86
    University of Pennsylvania, 62, 91
    University of Vienna, 113
    University of Washington School of Medicine, 97
    Wayne State University, 35
Urethra, lesions in, 103
Uric acid, 103
Urination, burning upon, 39, 103, 109
Urogenital cancer, 68

Vaccines, 17, 81-82, 93
    principle behind, 118
Vagina, sores on, 41
Vanadium 143
Varicella-zoster virus, 21-22

INDEX

JACKSON LIBRARY – LANDER UNIV.
RC147.H6 F73 1982 c.1   CIRC
Herpes : a complete guide to relief & reassurance /

3 6289 001042909

RC 147 .H6 F73 1982   346022

Freudberg, Frank.

Herpes : a complete guide to
relief & reassurance /

JUL 3 1984	NOV 6 1986	APR 0 8 1996
JUL 2 4 1984	NOV 2 5 1986	APR 24 1996
DEC 4 1984	JUN 2 8 '88	FEB 0 1 1999
APR 2 3 1985	SEP 1 2 1989	
JUL 3 0 1985	APR 1 4 1992	
AUG 9 1985	MAR 3 0 1993	
JAN 2 8 1986	FEB 2 3 1994	
FEB 2 7 1986	NOV 2 7 1994	
SEP 3 0 1986	052295	

CARD REMOVED

Jackson Library
Lander College
Greenwood, SC   29646